# A Better Way to Practice Dentistry

# Dr. Timothy Leary
# Dr. Michael Schuster

*Cover Art by Dr. Charlie Dingman*

*The cover art depicts our struggle to overcome challenges, and our need for others to reach out and help us.*

*Jonathan Livingston Seagull, from the book by Richard Bach, is in the upper right corner. Jonathan represents anyone who refuses to be ordinary. He, like all who seek to be extraordinary, learns there is a price to pay for becoming the best version of yourself. Jonathan became a symbol of the Schuster Center because our purpose was to help each person we engaged become the best they can become. Occasionally, we gave out a "Jonathan" pin to supporters and advocates of the Schuster Center.*

*We live in a culture that honors excellence in athletics but does its best to keep the rest of us in mediocrity. Jonathan was banished from his community when he tried to tell others that there was something more to life than scrambling for food and competing with each other for survival. The Jonathan story is for all of us.*

*- Mike Schuster*

# Testimonials to the Schuster Method

*"OBI, has had many of your former students enroll in our courses. Happily, I discovered that all of them have been well prepared financially to seek practice maturity. This training enabled OBI to help them upgrade their diagnostic and treatment skills. You certainly have our endorsement because your purpose, like ours, puts the patient first and is dedicated to help dentists provide the highest quality of service for their patients."*

- Charles R. Wold, DMD, Director, Orognathic Bioesthetics, International, (OBI)

*"We have had many orthodontists go through our two-year comprehensive program and become technically proficient, but few have been able to adequately integrate this material into their practice, reduce their volume, and raise their fees. The ones that have gone through your program at the Schuster Center have all been able to integrate our approach and prosper, thanks to your program.*

*"I would highly recommend your program to any orthodontist or a general dentist that truly wishes to learn how to have a high-quality, low volume, income generating practice. There is no one else out there who concentrates on building the "quality" practice. God bless you and keep up the good work! Also, my personal thanks for all you have done for our people who have gone through your program."*

- Ronald H. Roth, DDS, MS, FACD, FICD, Clinical Professor of Orthodontics, University of Detroit/Mercy, University of the Pacific, Diplomate American Board of Orthodontics.

*"Thank you for the excellent training you have offered to our FACE graduates. Our efforts to turn out the best technical dentists in the world are truly enhanced by the philosophy and excellence of your training program.*

*"Those who have graduated from both FACE and your program have more easily achieved their goals. It is gratifying to know during a time in dentistry when the practitioner is offered courses that promise success through less than ethical means, there are programs like yours. Your programs help the quality-oriented dentist achieve not only financial freedom, but also a life of dignity and professional satisfaction."*

- Thomas F. Basta, D.D.S., Director, Foundation for Advanced
Continuing Education (FACE)

# Dedication

This book is dedicated to Lizette, Joan, Carol, and the dental team members I've worked with over my career. I found the quality of dental care provided is proportional to the quality of the relationship between the doctor and the team.

And to Mrs. Barth, my high school English teacher, and my father, William Leary Jr., who both challenged me and nurtured my interest in writing.

*- Tim Leary*

# Contents

Dedication ................................................................. iii

Preface ...................................................................... 1

Introduction .............................................................. 4

Part One  How The Model Was Developed ................... 9

Chapter One A Dreadful Beginning ......................... 10

Chapter Two Health Is First ................................... 25

Chapter Three  Controlling Money ......................... 32

Chapter Four  Organization & Controlling Time ...... 45

Chapter Five  A Philosophy of Excellence and Professional Service .... 58

Chapter Six  The Power Shift .................................. 71

Part Two  How I Shared the Model and Created the First Business School for Dentists ................................... 78

Chapter Seven  Teaching at the Pankey Institute ....... 79

Chapter Eight  The Schuster Model for Practice Success .... 90

Chapter Nine The Power of Purpose ....................... 101

Afterward ................................................................. 119

Part Three  Schuster Center Alumni Professional Biographies ........... 136

Chapter Ten Dr. Robin Steely ................................ 137

Chapter Eleven Dr. John Korolewski ...................... 146

Chapter Twelve Dr. Sue Vetter .............................. 157

Chapter Thirteen Dr. Mike Edwards, CEO of the Schuster Center ...... 169

Chapter Fourteen Raymond Hsu, DDS, MAGD, LLSR ...... 185

Chapter Fifteen Dr. TJ Bolt .................................. 199

Chapter Sixteen Dr. Sharon Dickerson .................... 208

Chapter Seventeen Dr. Fred Arnold ........................ 221

Chapter Eighteen Dr. Mary Isaacs .......................... 234

Chapter Nineteen Dr. Mike Robichaux ................................. 251

Chapter Twenty Dr. Jack King................................................ 265

Chapter Twenty-One Dr. Jim Sandlin ................................... 281

Chapter Twenty-Two Dr. Ivette Rodriguez............................ 291

Chapter Twenty-Three Dr. Charlie Dingman........................ 302

Chapter Twenty-Four Dr. Eniko Loud .................................. 312

Chapter Twenty-Five Dr. Peyton Cunningham..................... 324

Chapter Twenty-Six Dr. Cree Hamilton............................... 335

Chapter Twenty-Seven Dr. Scott McKinney........................ 350

Chapter Twenty-Eight Dr. Timothy Leary ........................... 368

Appendix 1 Power Shift ........................................................ 391

Appendix 2 The 7 Driving Forces of your Practice............. 401

Appendix 3 Reading List....................................................... 403

Curriculum Vitae Dr. Michael Schuster .............................. 415

Curriculum Vitae, Dr. Tim Leary......................................... 417

*The Ascent*

*Grab hold ,*

*And take this hand that*

*Reaches out to you.*

*Look up*

*Into my eyes;*

*My spirit*

*Cries out to you:*

*Friendship is my thought.*

*Let us climb*

*The jagged cliffs of life*

*And fight the ascent of*

*Opposition together.*

*If I can lift you today,*

*You will look back*

*And grab the hands of a thousand more.*

*That is the way*

*The Great Spirit would have it!*

*- Howard Rainer, Native American Poet*

# Preface

Many people have influenced my thinking, but no one more than my students, as I witnessed their lives improve. I met most dentists in a state of discontent, distress, disharmony, confusion, low energy, and without control of money or time. When I met them, they were distrustful, resentful, angry, and often depressed. These are symptoms of negative energy. They had negative energy because they weren't satisfying their basic needs. Their outward behavior was not congruent with their inner core values. Within a year or less, I observed dramatic transformations in their lives and their practices. As they gained control of money and time and organized their practice and life, I saw them feel more alive, more positive, and more hopeful. They were achieving their goals and aspirations. They evolved from scarcity thinking to a world view of abundance. They were learning and growing by applying key strategies they learned at the Schuster Center. Their lives improved dramatically, as mine had. They were happier, healthier, and established meaningful relationships at home and at the office. They experienced a transformation, a change in thinking, behavior, and results.

This book has a bold promise. It will help you create a better practice and a better life. The book includes stories of dentists like you. The message of the stories is simple yet profound. This is also a book about discovering a method that can transform your life and the patients you work with. You are the architect of your life. You live in two worlds: the world you have and the world you hope for. We believe by reading our book, your thinking will begin to shift. You will become different than you were before you read it. If your practice and your life aren't what you hoped it would be, then reading our stories will give you hope.

We are dentists like you. We decided to share our stories because we believe good news should be shared. You'll probably relate to a few stories more than others. Within my story were discoveries that changed my life and then changed the lives of many dentists, their teams, and their patients. This book is about discovery and how I used what I learned to change my practice and my life for the better. Other stories relate how dentists applied the same principles to create the practice and life they wanted. The key is motivation. You get what you want if you have the desire and take action to get it.

*"Whatever ye want, oh discontented man; step up, pay the price, and take it!"*

*- Napolean Hill*

The source of invention and creation is not only looking for something better but discontent with what you have. It was true for me and true for others who will share their stories. Something must be wrong before we seek what is right. Creating an extraordinary life comes from dissatisfaction with living an ordinary life. All truths must be lived before they are shared. This is why each story is important. Each story reveals two lives: the life we had and the life we created.

My story has two parts as I had two parallel careers. I practiced dentistry for fifty-two years, and I taught clinical, management, and humanistic dentistry for forty-eight years. **Part I: Chapters 1-6** are how the model was developed. **Part II Chapters 7-9** are how I shared the model and created the Business School for Dentists, including:

- Thirty-five years and more than 1,000 days of speaking throughout the US, Canada, Puerto Rico, and Europe. Ten million miles of travel.

- Twenty-two books, programs, and manuals.

- Forty years of learning, applying, and teaching at the Schuster Center.

-  The creation of advanced programs of Mastery, CEO, Leadership, and Performance Coach.

*- Dr. Michael Schuster*

# Introduction

The dental profession is experiencing a hostile takeover. Big business is grabbing profit and control at the expense of doctor success and patient health. Young dentists are drowning in debt and suffering in high-volume commodity practices controlled by corporations or the insurance industry. Dental patients are trapped in repair-focused disease management. Patient health has become subordinate to business profit for corporate shareholders.

This book is an antidote to the nasty business that has infected health care. It offers hope and renewal of the time honored, professional relationship cherished by doctors and patients. It gets health care right by making the best interests of the patient primary and business interests secondary. This book shows dentists a path, a step-by-step process, to create a wonderful life and practice. It shows how to make a dramatic difference in your life and the lives of your patients and team members. The experience of thousands of dentists proves the Schuster Model works. It delivers the promise IF the dentist DOES the work. Thus, the real question becomes—will the dentist do the work?

The book is divided into three parts. **Parts One and Two,** written by Dr. Michael Schuster, is his account of his extraordinary career. Dr. Schuster spent his life studying with giants of the dental profession, innovators of patient-centered relationships, and leaders in business development. We learn how he built his dental practice and became a master dentist. His practice success attracted dentists from around the country to understand his philosophy, methods, and systems. We learn how and why he developed the first Business School for dentists and team members, The Center for Professional Development (CPD,) later renamed the Schuster Center (SC.) He practiced full-time for the first 25 years, then he practiced two days a week for 25 years and devoted more time to teaching, speaking, and writing about health-centered, patient-centered dental care. He spoke to thousands of dentists and team members, and he was a keynote speaker at all the major national dental meetings.

Learn how Dr. Schuster, through study, training, and experience, created a model for practice success—the Schuster Model. It's a practice blueprint incorporating sound business principles, modern learning theory, motivational coaching, and practical strategies that can be adapted to your personal style and preferences. The model focuses on health, professional service, clinical excellence, strong team dynamics, honest communication, fiscal responsibility, and practice philosophy. It's not surprising that many Schuster Center graduates, doctors, and staff members became leading teachers in dentistry. Some developed courses of clinical excellence, while others teach about team and practice development.

**Part Three** is my contribution, collating many hours of interviews into professional memoirs. Each chapter includes an inspiring story from a dentist whose practice and personal life were transformed by the Schuster Model. Most doctors found better profit and gained control of money. They got organized and reduced staff discord. They found relief from stress and career burnout, and they renewed their joy for dentistry. Nearly all were able to slow down and find richer, deeper, caring relationships with patients, staff, family, and the people in their lives. Most significantly increased their practice profit, wealth, and freedom.

All the Schuster Center graduates significantly improved patient acceptance of necessary treatment and complete care dentistry. High-pressure sales favored in the business world are replaced with goal-directed coaching methods that help patients make good decisions. It's a pull strategy, not manipulation or pushing patients into treatment. It's NOT what dentists are taught by consultants and other management groups. Instead, through awareness and learning about health and disease problems, patients come to ask for the treatment they need.

Schuster Center dentists pay off debt and achieve financial freedom in ten to fifteen years. Most no longer need to work for a living. Dentistry becomes a hobby, not a burden. Pressure and stress are reduced as dentists slow down and create more meaningful relationships with staff and patients. They work less at a relaxed pace because they enjoy caring for patients, enjoy working with loyal staff, and enjoy the type of dentistry they provide.

This book has the perspective of dentists practicing dentistry. However, the strategies within the model can be applied successfully to any service-based business. Here's just a few:

- Clarifying your values and what is most important to you.

- A written philosophy to filter decision-making and create the future you prefer.

- Understanding that your practice (business) exists primarily to serve the client.

- Percentage budgeting, overhead control, profit planning, and cost-based fee setting.

- A new client process that engages each person in forming specific reasons and goals for themselves.

- Systems based management for increasing effectiveness and reducing stress.

- Client qualification and prioritizing your mix of services.

- Leveraging the 80/20 principle to create a win/win environment for clients and the professional team.

Dr. Schuster and many of his clients lived the hero's journey. They were each dissatisfied with the practice they had and made a commitment to create a better practice and life. The method Dr. Schuster created and lived helps you learn how to leave the ordinary world of mainstream, disease care, repair dentistry. Answer the call of the road less travelled. Wander in the forest with us as you discover a better way to practice and live. Find magic with a professional doctor/patient relationship, systems management, team development, and health-centered care. Slay the dragons of insurance restrictions, and corporate business control. Learn how to get on the path of financial freedom, time freedom, and relationship freedom. Then, enjoy the rest of your career with optimum profits, meaningful work, and fulfillment with your patients and team.

*- Tim Leary*

# Part One

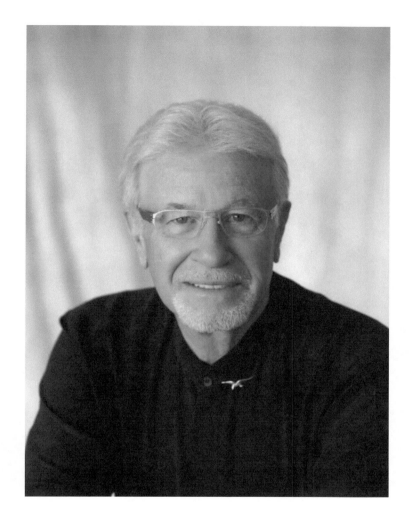

# How The Model Was Developed

# Chapter One
# A Dreadful Beginning

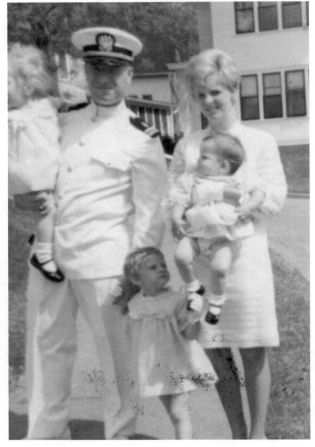

*Dr Schuster, wife JoAnne, and daughters Dianne, Cathy, and Christy*

*"There's nothing wrong with dentistry, but there is something wrong with the way you are practicing it!"*

*- Dr. Robert Barkley*

We were driving home to Dyersville, Iowa, after a movie in Dubuque. The pain in my chest was severe. I was having trouble breathing, and I was frightened. My wife, and a nurse, was with me. She thought I was having a heart attack, so we drove straight to the hospital. After a series of tests, it was determined that I had a bleeding duodenal bleeding ulcer, not a heart attack.

There I was, in a hospital bed, at age 28! My three young daughters came to visit me in the hospital. "What's the matter with Daddy?" they asked. Something was alarmingly wrong, but what? The doctors kept me in the hospital for a week to monitor my health.

My father, a college professor, sensed that there was something seriously wrong. He gave me two books to read: <u>Motivation and Personality</u> by Abraham Maslow and <u>Individual Psychology</u> by Alfred Adler.

I remember something Adler wrote, *"Act as if, and you will become it!"* Adler's statement became a mantra for my life. Maslow addressed his theory of motivation based on the satisfaction of human needs. Health, he wrote, requires that a person be able to satisfy their basic human needs. If a person can't satisfy their basic needs, he will be distressed, upset, angry, depressed, and the body will respond in some visible way. It seemed Maslow had written his book for me. My distress and despair had brought on physical illness, and now I had a bleeding ulcer. My body rejected the dental practice I had.

I went to work when I was just eleven years old. My parents were teachers. We lived in Kirkwood, a suburb of St. Louis. On a teacher's salary, there was little money left after paying for our home and food. If I was to have anything extra, I had to pay for it. I started caddying at Westborough Country Club, which was a six-mile walk one way from our house. I worked so I could buy a bicycle rather than walk the twelve miles every time I caddied. Later, I bought my own cars and clothes. Little was given to me growing up.

My parents raised me to believe I was special and had something important to do with my life. They had two boys before me and one boy born after. They all died of Erythroblastosis Fetalis, known as Rh incompatibility. I was the only son who survived. Today, those infants would be immediately transfused and would have lived. It's hard for me to imagine the pain my mom and dad felt. I remember taking my mother to see the movie Titanic years ago. At an emotional point in the film, she turned to me and said, *"I can't cry anymore. I wept all my tears after Steven died."* Steven was my parent's last son who didn't survive. Patrick and Timothy before me and Steven after me. All died in childbirth. That's why they instilled everything they could into me. They supported whatever I attempted, even when I messed up. They provided me with the finest education and support available. My dad, previously an officer in the Army, was a strict disciplinarian. My mother, a positive thinker, was the best cheerleader I ever had. She believed in me more than I believed in myself. She infused me with her "Positive Irish Spirit."

My parents and grandparents were all highly educated and successful in their chosen professions. There was an expectation of excellence and service that both my mom and dad instilled in me. They said, "Whatever you do, do it the best you can." My parents were both devout Christians who walked their talk. It had a profound effect on me. They instilled respect and reverence for each human being within me. My mom often said to me,

*"What you are is God's gift to you. What you do with it is your gift to God."*

We lived in Dubuque, Iowa. I worked at the Dubuque Golf and Country Club. I had other jobs as well. I unloaded box cars for Bly Lumber Company. I sold ice cream to kids and mothers. I sold and carried beef for the Dubuque Packing Company. I went to college in Dubuque and worked at the Country Club from 10-2 every day, tending bar. I also worked weekends for parties, weddings, and other events. My college tuition was pro bono because my dad was faculty at Loras College. I played baseball in high school and college.

By the time I went to dental school, I had saved more than $100,000, which went a lot farther in 1963 than it does today. I graduated from Loras College in three years. I was accepted to several dental schools, but I chose Marquette. I was married after my first year in dental school. I didn't work the first eighteen months of dental school. Midway through my second year I worked full-time as a bartender at the Black Kettle Restaurant in Milwaukee, and I continued full-time until graduation. I had a great experience working for Dorothy Edwards at the Black Kettle. She taught me how to care for employees. My wife, an RN, often worked double shifts at Milwaukee County Hospital. We paid for all my dental school costs, plus living costs, except the last two-quarters of tuition. We borrowed $7,000 from my uncle to pay the last of my tuition.

The US Navy had an Ensign 1925 program for dental students. I enrolled and earned four years of Naval Reserve time while in dental school. The Navy paid no dental school expenses. I graduated at the top of my class clinically. I had a good experience in dental school, though some of the instructors tried to make it difficult. If a student had good hands, they were pretty much left alone. Several of the clinical instructors at Marquette were the best I have ever had.

After graduation from Marquette, I went on active duty for two years at Willow Grove Naval Air Station. My assignment was operative dentistry. On Fridays, I'd spend my time studying and preparing for private practice. Captain Bill Crolius, retired and then clinical coordinator at Temple Dental School, asked me if I was interested in teaching part-time. I said yes to the opportunity, which opened a whole new world for me. I met many notable dentists, including D. Walter Cohen, Morten Amsterdam, Selzer and Bender, Bill Updegrave, Herman Corn, and Captain Bill Fetti.

I took many courses, but the most important was a week-long course at the Walter Reed Army Hospital. Each day, we had a different instructor with a different agenda.

Day 1: Jay Siebert, DDS, MS. <u>Conservative Periodontal Therapy</u>

Day 2: D. Walter Cohn, DDS, MS. <u>Periodontal Surgical Therapy</u>

Day 3. Harold Loe, a researcher. <u>Bacterial plaque and the causes of Periodontal Disease and Dental Decay</u>

Day 4: Robert Barkley, DDS. <u>Dental Disease Control Therapy - Helping patients learn to control dental disease.</u>

Day 5: Bob Cassidy, PhD, <u>Dental Behavior Science - The challenges of helping patients change and take responsibility for themselves.</u>

I didn't know that the week at Walter Reed Hospital would alter the direction of my practice and my life. The emphasis of my education and training at Marquette was on the treatment of dental disease. Little attention was given to understanding the causes or prevention of dental disease. The week at Walter Reed was my first exposure to understanding, controlling, and preventing the causes of oral disease. My mind was opened to something totally different. My thinking began to change, but I didn't know what to do with what I was learning.

I completed my tour in the Navy and moved my family to Dyersville, Iowa. Today, Dyersville is known for the movie **Field of Dreams**. I had been recruited by Bud Ross, a civic leader in Dyersville. He promised a new Medical Arts Building would be completed by the time I arrived. When we got to Dyersville, the Medical Arts Building was just being built, so I had no place to practice. What was I to do? There I was with my wife and three little girls, ages four, three, and two, and no job or income.

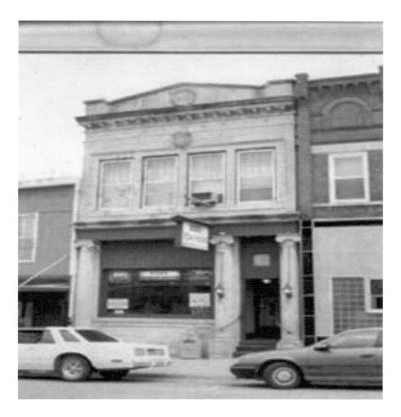

*First dental office, second floor, Dyersville, Iowa*

Dr. Walter Barry, a local dentist, had retired six months before we arrived. He vacated his office and left his old, worn-out equipment. Old, wooden steps led up to his second-story office above a restaurant. Don (Scoop) Everest of Patterson Dental Supply company persuaded Dr. Barry to sell me his equipment but not the patient records. I paid $1,000 for his worn-out equipment.

I acquired an old stand-up Ritter pump-up chair, one high-speed handpiece, and old equipment that broke down on a regular basis. However, it was a place to start. We rented our home, and I was broke, having used my savings for dental school.

I thought I was prepared for private practice, but I was in for a rude awakening. Dyersville was a denture town. How was I to know that? Farmers would bring their 18-21-year-old sons to my office for the removal of all their teeth and replacement with dentures. "Let's get it over with," they would say. I was shocked! Who would take out a mouthful of healthy teeth?

People used me for emergency care. Often, at night, someone would knock on my bedroom window and wake me up to relieve the pain of their toothache or abscess. They knew the exact room I slept in! A famous physician in Dyersville suggested that people get all their teeth out so they could control arthritis. The ignorance was alarming. I refused to take out teeth that could be saved, which made me unpopular.

The practice was nothing like what I expected. What I had pictured was the opposite of my daily experience. Money was not the problem. I was making more money in one month than I made in a year in the Navy. But I hated it. Yet, I didn't know how to change it. I was so upset, in such turmoil, that I ended up in the hospital with a bleeding ulcer. That was the first time in my life when the invisible became visible to me. The invisible, emotional, and mental distress expressed itself visibly in the form of a bleeding ulcer!

Today, I realize there are two kinds of problems: visible ones and invisible ones. Even though I was saving $10,000 a month, I hated it. You might be thinking, he's making money and saving money; what's the problem with that? Something was missing to feel as negative as I did about my practice. I was achieving outward success but found myself struggling to create meaningful, trusting relationships with my patients. What I experienced wasn't what I had worked for all those nights and years. No amount of money could take the place of hating my practice. I learned that if I wasn't happy in my work, I sure wouldn't be happy at home.

Clearly, being unhappy at work affected the rest of my life and my health as well. I wasn't the father I wanted to be. I wasn't the husband I needed to be. I was angry, upset, and even outraged at what I was experiencing in my practice. I was getting negative feedback from patients, but I didn't know how to cope with it or change it.

The truth is, I was lost. I had worked my butt off for more than thirteen years, four years in high school, three years in college, and four years of dental school, plus the Navy for two more years. Now, I didn't even want to go to work. How could this happen to me?

While in the hospital, I did a lot of thinking. My life slowed down, and I read and reflected. The first couple of days, I considered quitting dentistry. Was this my future in dentistry? Was I doomed to be angry and unhappy working with people who didn't trust or respect me and people who resented paying for dental care? Was this health care-- repeated emergencies and destroying people's mouths? Was this normal? Was this how I was supposed to practice? Was I falling into the customary path in dentistry?

Other than emergency care, patients rarely accepted my recommendations for treatment. They didn't believe corrective treatment would last. Their previous experience was that treatment seldom lasted more than a few years, and it was a waste of money. So, they waited until the pain or infection was intolerable. I was busy pushing them into treatment. I had failed to discover what they really wanted.

An incident occurred that pushed me over the edge. One day, I was examining an eighteen-year-old boy with his father next to me. We took radiographs first, and then I placed them on the view box so we could see them together. I examined the boy's mouth and recorded my findings in his chart. I noted considerable decay with red marks. As I finished the upper arch, the father stopped me and said, "That's enough, isn't it?" I must have had a puzzled look on my face as I said to him, "What do you mean, that's enough?" He said, "It seems to me you've found enough to keep yourself busy for a while?" I lost my cool. His remark showed ignorance and distrust. I'm not proud of what I did next. I grabbed the father, escorted him down the old wooden steps, and told him, "Never come back!" My overreaction revealed months of pent-up frustration and anger.

Had I spent years working day and night to end up watching people lose their teeth? I knew what I was experiencing was wrong. I knew I didn't like it, and I couldn't continue to do it. However, I didn't know what to change or how.

Whatever I was doing wasn't suitable for my patients either. They rejected me. Didn't trust me. Didn't like me. I hit a wall early, and I've been forever grateful that I did. I was young, eager, and motivated to do something meaningful with my life. That was instilled in me as a child. Had I not resisted early, I might have gotten used to it and settled on the well-worn path of sickness care. As I reflected on my emotional state, I realized that the days I spent with Harold Loe, Robert Barkley, and Bob Cassidy changed something in me. They planted a seed in me that began to grow. The experience at Walter Reed gave me a glimpse of a different way to practice. Barkley made the biggest impression on me, and I began to conceptualize a different picture of dental practice. I remember clearly Barkley saying several times, "When a barn is on fire, what should you do first? Start to repair the roof or put out the fire?" I was trapped in patching, even destroying the barn, without any effort to put out the fire.

I was at a loss, so I called Barkley on the phone and explained my predicament. I remember the words he spoke. His initial experience in practice had been similar. Barkley spoke very directly. He told me, "There's nothing wrong with dentistry, but there is something wrong with the way you are practicing it."

I was lost because I had no plan and no guidelines. I fell into a crisis because I lacked a purpose for what I was doing. Stated another way, my purpose was invisible. Something inside of me was saying, what you are doing isn't right! I didn't know what to say to patients. I didn't know how to get them interested in keeping their teeth. I didn't know what each day, each week, each month would bring. Previously, I had some sort of plan. Study to pass tests. Work to pay the bills and put food on the table. Pay for my education. Everything had been laid out for me, and I worked the plan that was made for me. Even the Navy had plenty of structure. Now, I was fighting to stay alive.

In all the jobs I had growing up, the people I worked for were happy with my work. I showed up early, worked hard, and went the extra mile. Kids and their mothers were glad to buy ice cream from me during a summer job. Leo Bly was pleased that I'd work my tail off unloading lumber from box cars. People were happy to pay for drinks at the country club. I worked hard at the Dubuque Golf and Country Club and later at the Dubuque Packing Company. The patrons of the Black Kettle were happy to pay me for the drinks they loved. My experience in the Navy and at Temple Dental School was positive.

However, my practice in Dyersville put me into the hospital. I was distressed, sick, and lost, wondering what had happened.

Today, many years later, I realize my practice was focused on what my patients needed but didn't want. I wasn't prepared to deal with negative mindsets. Why were people telling me they wanted healthy teeth removed? Why did they only want emergency care? Why was I having so much difficulty connecting with people? What were they really telling me? I didn't know how to communicate with my patients. I didn't know how to get their attention and help them think differently. I simply couldn't cope. While in the hospital, I began to develop a different perspective. What Harold Loe, Robert Barkley, and Robert Cassidy said kept coming to mind. I had been following a traditional, well-worn path of dentistry. I was treating the problems and the effects of disease, but not the causes of disease.

Seeking answers to these problems changed the direction of my practice and my life. As my thinking changed, my life and practice changed. I was in the process of being transformed.

Through study and reflection I came to understand my patients really wanted three things. They wanted:

- No dentistry or as little as possible.

- To spend as little money on their teeth as possible.

- Yet, they wanted to be pain-free, comfortable, to speak clearly, and to eat what they wanted to eat.

What did I learn?

- I learned that when I was behaving in conflict with my values, I had a physical reaction. I got sick.

- I learned to ask questions and seek people who could help me.

# Chapter Two
# Health Is First

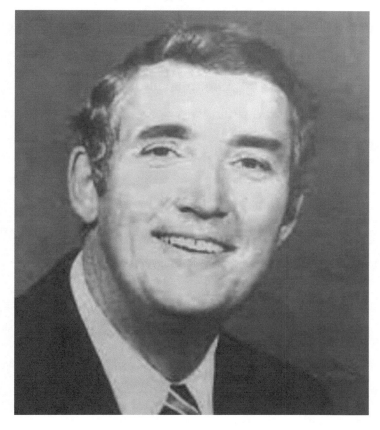

*Dr. Robert Barkley*

*"Mike, you've been too focused on the visible problem, the effects of disease, and the treatment of disease rather than on the cause of disease."*

*Dr. Robert Barkley*

Once I got clear on what I believed my patients really wanted, then my mindset changed. What if I could establish a practice focused on helping patients have as little dentistry as possible, spend as little money on their teeth as possible, and allow them to be pain-free, infection-free, and able to eat and chew comfortably? If I could help them spend less money and have less (no) disease, then I'd be giving them exactly what they wanted. I began to see that I could do this with Barkley's guidance. One day with Barkley changed my perspective. He helped me to see something that was there but had been invisible to me. Barkley helped me understand why controlling dental disease (putting out the fire) must come before mechanical repair (shingling the roof.)

In Barkley's lecture, he stated he made a decision to never slick a patient (to take all their teeth out). Something clicked in my mind that he said in his lecture. "Your job is to save people's teeth, not take them out." He said, "Health, the control of dental disease, the prevention of dental disease, should always be first." I had to figure out a way to help people understand the causes of dental disease and help them believe they could prevent disease. He went on to say, "You've been too focused on the visible problem, the effects of disease, and the treatment of disease, rather than on the cause of disease." Barkley understood what I had been facing because he had faced the same thing in Macomb, Illinois. He became my life's first and most valuable professional role model and mentor.

We talked at least once a month for several years. Below are the actions I took:

- First, I wrote out my thirteen beliefs about dentistry.

- I wrote my purpose: *Help people keep their teeth for life!*

- Then, I wrote my philosophy, the beliefs and values that would guide my practice.

- I showed each new patient a series of photos I had taken of street people in Philadelphia who had lost all their teeth. I'd show four pictures (5 x 7) of street people and ask each patient, "How old do you think this person is?" They guessed at least twenty years older than each person really was. It was my first and earliest attempt to show what the loss of all teeth does to the face. It worked to a degree.

- The Dreadful Story is a pamphlet that shows the progression of periodontal disease and decay from health to tooth loss. Why the Dreadful Story? Because most people who go to the dentist don't understand the causes of dental disease and how to control it.

- I developed a set of slides to show the effect of bacteria on the gums and teeth.

- I made a pamphlet to show the path of destruction due to untreated dental decay and gum disease.

- I took facial and intra-oral photos of every patient.

- I showed patients pictures of health and pictures of disease.

- I was attempting to make the invisible (causes of disease) become visible in a personalized, understandable format.

- I also showed a photo of a patched, broken-down highway and a new concrete highway, and I would ask, "Which of these is most like your mouth?"

- I began to show educational film strips that Barkley had provided me.

- I began doing saliva tests on all children because decay was rampant in Dyersville.

- Later, I gave every new patient a copy of the book Human Lifestyling.

I read one page from the book to every new patient. It described the progressive decline of a patient, George Clemmons, who visits his doctor complaining of heartburn. The doctor ignores George's symptoms because nothing abnormal is found on his radiographs. However, five years later, George returns with a bleeding ulcer. The doctor says, "Now I can treat you. You have a disease." George's life is saved. Through the years of medical observation (some call it malpractice), waiting for his symptoms to blossom into a full-blown clinical disorder, little attention was paid to the many factors of George's life that led to the bleeding ulcer: what he ate, what he breathed, what happened to his muscles and what his energy flow was. The ulcer could have been prevented. When his first symptom appeared, George could have made some lifestyle changes. Although George was unaware of it, George didn't get a bleeding ulcer. George gave himself a bleeding ulcer. The same is true for a person who suffers a heart attack; he gives himself a heart attack. In most clinical diseases, a person's lifestyle determines to a large extent what he gives himself and how severely he has done so.

We began using a percentage scoring chart that Herman Corn had developed and showed me while I was in the Navy. We charted each patient's mouth for plaque and bleeding and gave them a percentage score for dental plaque and bleeding. Further, we started scoring plaque and bleeding on patients at every recall appointment.

I employed Beth Hunter, a hygienist who believed in disease control and preventive dentistry. Beth, Sharon Bartels, and Linda Recker were all important to the practice transformation.

Then, I made a bold promise. If a patient stayed in our Disease Control Program and kept all preventive appointments, they wouldn't have dental decay and gum disease again. They would keep their teeth for life. The one caveat to this was fractured or broken teeth.

Because I had an early meltdown and sought out Barkley's help when I was young and idealistic, my practice and life began to change. It was Barkley who gave me hope. He taught me a better way. He was doing it and knew the process to transform me and my practice. I began to share the causes of dental disease and how dental disease impacts people's lives with each patient.

But I'm sure of one thing. I was determined to find or make a better way. Faced with adversity and a major crisis, I could either give in and give up or find a new way, a better way to practice. I chose not to give in and give up. This was the most crucial first step in beginning my professional and personal transformation, but not the last.

**What did I learn from my early failure?**

I learned that I had no visible reference points to make decisions. I realized that if I wasn't happy at work, I sure wouldn't be happy at home. I learned that money in the bank didn't take the place of enjoyment and feeling worthwhile at work! I realized that I had to have a plan, a purpose, and guidelines to enable me to do what was valuable for me. I learned patients needed a purpose, guidelines, and direction as well.

Maslow developed his theory of human motivation by studying the healthiest people he could find. I was busy finding out what was wrong with patients. I didn't have a picture of a healthy mouth in my mind. I got trapped in reacting to the people's disease. I was trying to get patients to do something they didn't understand or want--more repair and more expense. I fell into the well-worn pattern of plugging holes. That's what I was taught in dental school, and that's what I'd done in the Navy. Patients knew more than I did, and they didn't like what was happening to them. What had been invisible to me before became crystal clear as I lay in the hospital bed. Without reading Maslow and having early experience with Barkley, I doubt I would have come to understand what had happened or why it happened.

I learned that the distress in my first sixteen months in practice was caused by me acting in conflict with my beliefs and values. I learned to make my beliefs and values visible by writing them out and using them as a guide for how to practice. I learned to share my beliefs and values with each patient in a visible way. Since that time, I have used my beliefs and my values as a guide for how to practice and how to live. They have never changed.

# Chapter Three
# Controlling Money

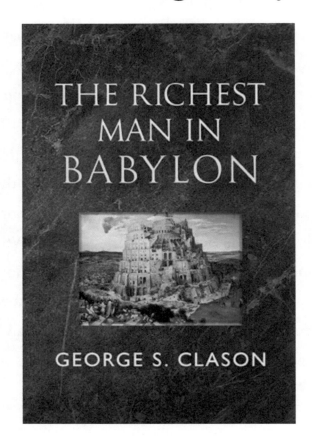

*"If you don't intend to live by the laws in this book, I don't want you for a client. I don't work with losers."*

*- Elliot Simon, Attorney*

I wasn't out of the woods yet. I still had much to learn. The first five years were the formative years of my professional life. After graduating from Marquette Dental School with a $7,000 debt, my uncle John Cain assisted in clearing it, which I repaid within my first year of practice. I was married during my first year and had two daughters, Catherine and Dianne, while both my wife and I worked full-time in the final three years of school. But I knew I was after something. I wanted a practice that I enjoyed.

I came out of the hospital with a picture of the practice I wanted to create. I still wasn't sure how to make it work. I knew I needed more help but from who, from where? I was saving money and am now planning for my new office in the Medical Arts Building in Dyersville. In my first full year in practice, I had managed to save $117,000, which was nearly as much as I made in a year in the Navy. I remember meeting with Tom Jenk, my attorney and accountant. Our conversation went like this. Tom said, "You had a good year." I said, "I think so." Then he said, "No, you had a really good year! In fact, your year was so good that you owe an additional $104,000 in Federal and State income tax!" Words can't describe how I felt. I was surprised, upset, and angry at the same time. Hard to believe?

If you go back to 1969 and look at the tax code, you will see that Federal Income tax was 70% of everything over $100,000 and

Iowa state tax was 8.5%. My office rent was $150. I employed one assistant at $450. My house rental cost $150. I had no debt repayments and no equipment payments, so all of my income was exposed to taxes. My gross income was around $17,000 a month, but my overhead had to be less than $3,000 a month. The rest was taxable income. I had no planning and no guidelines with money. I was making it and saving it, but Uncle Sam was taking the bulk of it.

I had worked long days to get through school, pay for school, move my family, and start a practice that I hated. Now, I felt like I was working for the government, and that made the whole thing even worse. But what was I to do about it?

I drove to Iowa City to see if I could teach part-time at Iowa Dental School. While teaching at Temple, I met many wonderful dentists and learned a great deal. I wanted to continue teaching and learning. There were no positions in the operative department, so they sent me to see Claude Fraleigh, the head of the Department of Periodontology. I told him of my interest in prevention and periodontal care. He offered me both a teaching position and the opportunity to become a part-time student in the Department of Periodontics at Iowa. I was at Iowa Dental School two days a week for three years. It was there that I met many highly motivated dentists like Steven Cooper, a periodontist from Davenport, Larry

34

Huber, a Prosthodontist, and others. In my second and third years of practice, I was in a gnathology study group with Niles Guichet. Eight of us, under Dr. Guichet's supervision and mentoring, completed a full mouth restoration. In the next year, Dr. Larry Huber guided us through two more full mouth reconstructions, step by step, stage by stage. After we completed our second year, we started the Northeast Iowa Gnathology Study Club. We met quarterly to go over cases with each other.

Writing this seems unreal. I was lucky, blessed, or destined. I'm not sure how to best describe my experience. My early frustration with my practice was relieved but was replaced by frustration with my tax situation. I was restoring the mouth of Dr. Sol Tabek, an Ophthalmologist from Dubuque. I described my frustration with my tax situation.

He referred me to Elliott Simon, his corporate attorney in Chicago. Elliott's specialty was setting up C-Corporations for highly taxed professionals. I'd been learning a lot about the science of dentistry but not much about managing money or practice management. I called Elliott and made an appointment. I drove to Chicago to meet him. We spoke for about an hour, and he gave me a book, which I'm looking at as I'm writing this. It has a gold leaf cover, The Richest Man in Babylon, by George S. Clason. He told me to read the book and come back for another appointment. We hadn't talked much about a C-Corporation, but we went over my tax issue. I went back in three weeks. We met at the Whitehall Hotel for lunch, which lasted until 4 PM.

We had an elegant lunch, and then he began talking about the Clason book. He underlined some key statements from the book. Here are a few:

*"This book of cures for lean purses has been termed a guide for financial understanding. That, indeed, is its purpose: to offer those who are ambitious for financial success an insight which will aid them to acquire money, to keep money, and to make their surpluses earn more money."*

*"If you have not acquired more than a bare existence in the years since youth, it is because you have either failed to learn the laws that govern the building of wealth, or else you failed to observe them."*

*"A part of all you earn is yours to keep. It should be not less than one-tenth, no matter how little you earn. It can be as much as you can afford. Pay yourself first. Do not buy from the clothes-maker and the sandal-maker more than you can pay out of the rest and still have enough for food and charity and penance to the gods."*

Elliot went through the book, page by page, with me and highlighted key statements with a yellow marker. This is what he underlined.

*THE FIRST CURE: Start thy purse to fattening.*

*For every ten coins thou place within thy purse, take out and use but nine. Thy purse will start to fatten at once, and its increasing weight will feel good in thy hand and bring satisfaction to your soul.*

I interpreted this to mean that I had to save 10% of whatever income I made.

*THE SECOND CURE: Control thy expenses.*

*Now, I will tell thee an unusual truth about men and sons of men. It is this: That what each of us calls our necessary expenses will always grow to meet our incomes unless we protest to the contrary. All men are burdened with more desires than they can gratify. Because of my wealth, thinketh thou that I may gratify every desire? Budget thy necessary expenses. Though not the one-tenth that is fattening your purse. Let this be thy great desire that is being fulfilled. Keep working with thy budget, keep adjusting it to help thee. Make it thy first assistant in defending a fattening purse.*

I recognized I needed to budget my expenses and outgo. If I was to control money in my life, then I had to have a way to do it. That led me to percentage budgeting.

*THE THIRD CURE: Make thy gold multiply.*

*This, then, is the third cure for a lean purse: to put each coin to laboring that it may reproduce its kind even as the flocks of the field and help bring to thee income, a stream of wealth that shall flow constantly into thy purse.*

I needed to invest the money I saved so it would grow and compound over time. Later, I read that Einstein stated, *"Compound interest is the eighth wonder of the world."* Some question whether Einstein said it, but there is little doubt about the power of compound interest.

*THE FOURTH CURE: Guard your treasures from loss.*

As Elliot took me through the book, he gave several examples of what people fail to do and why they get into trouble. He said several times. The key to getting ahead is to find the right people to help you. Every successful person he'd ever met had found the right people and followed their guidance. It was vital that I learn how to make my investments profitable and keep them safe and secure.

*THE FIFTH CURE: Make thy dwelling a profitable investment.*

*No man's family can fully enjoy life unless they have a plot of ground wherein children can play on the clean earth and where the wife may raise not only blossoms but good rich herbs to feed her family.*

I was never sure how this cure would impact my life. I believed that it was important to live in a house we enjoyed, and that was a welcome place for friends and family. In my lifetime, I've owned several homes and made money on every one of them.

*THE SIXTH CURE: Insure a future income.*

*Therefore, do I say that it behooves a man in the days to come, when he is no longer young, to make preparations for his family should he no longer be with them to comfort and support them. The man who, because of his understanding of the laws of wealth, acquireth a growing surplus should give thought to those future days. He should plan certain investments or provisions that may endure safely for many years yet will be available when the time arrives, which he so wisely anticipated.*

This became an important guideline in my life. I understood there will come a time in my life when I no longer desire to work. It is vital I have a plan and a budget for both income and expenses when I stop working.

At this point, Elliot began to outline how he would help me. He related the importance of converting a significant part of the taxes I was paying into a tax-deferred savings and investment plan.

It was at this point that he began to lay out a plan for a Defined Pension Plan and a Profit-Sharing plan. He outlined various tax laws that I knew nothing about and how we would use these government-approved laws to aid me in creating wealth.

Converting tax dollars into a savings plan for my family sounded very good to me. I liked the idea of reducing my taxes, but I liked the idea of using the money I had already earned for investments for my family. I didn't fully understand it then, but now I understand the importance of starting a tax-deferred savings plan is perhaps the best reason to own a business.

*THE SEVENTH CURE: Increase your ability to earn.*

*Preceding accomplishment must be desired. Thy desires must be strong and definite.*

*The more wisdom we know, the more we may earn. The man who seeks to learn more of his craft shall be richly rewarded. The seventh and last remedy for a lean purpose is to cultivate thy own powers, to study and become wiser, to become more skillful, to act as to respect thyself.*

I learned to focus on what I would give to enable the life I wanted to live. I knew I wanted to make a difference in the lives of my patients. I wanted to learn more so that I could create ever-increasing value for my patients.

This meeting in Chicago in May of 1970 was pivotal in my life experience and in my family's experience. I found sound principles to build my financial future around. I've kept this in mind my entire life. I learned three simple guidelines regarding money that shaped my experience with money.

- First, you have to earn it.

- Second, learn how to keep it.

- Third, learn where to put it so you don't lose it.

At the time, I was making money, but I wasn't keeping it. I was paying far too much in income tax. My attorney/accountant, Tom Jenk, didn't spend any time with me in preparation or planning. I simply got to the end of the year and paid taxes on the money I had made.

I didn't want to spend my life reacting. I didn't want to react to the patient's disease or react to the loss of money because of poor planning. I believed my family and I deserved better.

At the end of the meeting, Elliot said something to me that I vividly remember. He said, ***"If you don't intend to live by the laws in this book, I don't want you for a client. I don't work with losers."*** Wow, what a powerful statement. Fortunately, I found another guide who didn't mince words. He was telling me, in no uncertain terms, that to win with money, I had to play by certain rules. The rules are clearly spelled out in a simple but powerful manner in <u>The Richest Man in Babylon.</u> I agreed. I not only wanted to win with money, but I wanted to win in life. How could I win in life without winning with money? Now, I had money guidelines to live by, but I had never guidelined with money before.

My parents rarely talked about money. It was clear, however, that they didn't have much of it. I remember, as a young child living in Kirkwood, occasionally, we'd go to Webster Groves to a small restaurant for dinner on Sunday. My Dad would point to what I could order on the menu. It was always the cheapest thing on the menu. I made a promise to myself that one day when I went out to eat, I wouldn't focus on the price.

Prior to starting a practice, I had worked hard and saved for books, for a car, and for school. That had gotten me to this point, but it wasn't enough to take us into the future. I'm repeating this for a reason. Elliot told me that if I didn't intend to live by the principles in Richest Man in Babylon, he didn't want me for a client. This was the second time I reached out for help. Both Barkley and Simon were direct in their approach. Most people are begging for work, bending over backward to get your business. Elliott Simon laid down the gauntlet at the beginning of our relationship. In fact, he was defining how we'd work together, and he gave me the reasons, the principles, and the rules of how I was going to control money and create wealth.

We worked together. I formed a C-Corporation and set up a Defined Pension Plan, which allowed me to set aside a significant amount of money each year and defer the taxes. That meeting and my commitment to live by the principles Clason had laid out enabled me to achieve a net worth of nearly 3 million dollars by age thirty-nine. Creating abundance and wealth at that age provided me with options and opportunities I wouldn't have had otherwise.

**What did I learn?**

I learned that to get ahead, I had to surround myself with the best accountants, tax advisors, and attorneys I could find. I learned to lay out the ground rules of a relationship and the reasons for it directly and clearly with patients. Elliott Simon taught me an important lesson on how to establish a relationship with a new client.

Elliott was a great role model.

I began to share three things with every new patient:

- I want to do worthwhile work.

- I want to enjoy my time in the office.

- I want to make a profit.

As I write this, looking back at my life, I'm convinced of this. Whenever I had a problem, one that mattered to me, I sought out the help and guidance of the best person I could find in their field. Then,

I took action. I followed their advice. I know today that both are key to success: finding the right people to help and acting on what is learned.

# Chapter Four
# Organization & Controlling Time

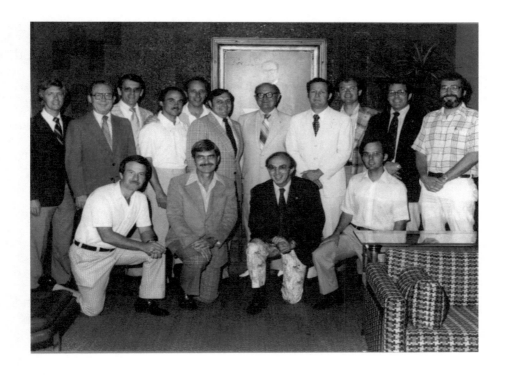

*Dr. LD Pankey and the original Cadre at the Pankey Institute*

*"Percentage budgeting with money and time led me to the realization that Less Is More."*

*- Dr. Michael Schuster*

My second year in practice was another year of searching. A year of seeking solutions to the problems I was experiencing. But with new hope and confidence, I felt positive. Patient problems, treatment acceptance problems, and patient resistance problems had put me in the hospital with an ulcer. Thankfully, with Barkley's help, I discovered a purpose and a vision for my practice. These were vital first steps. The tax problem was mostly resolved over the next year.

Now, since I was also teaching, I'd drive to Iowa City two days a week, ninety-five miles each way. While driving, I'd listen to audiotapes. I wore out two sets of tapes listening to James Neuman's Release Your Brakes. I began reading As A Man Thinketh, by James Allen every day. Teaching, listening to tapes, and commitment to reading changed my perspective. I became more interested in human behavior and motivation. Why were some people motivated and others not? Why did some people take action and others did not?

In December of 1969 I flew to Phoenix to take a seminar with Omer Reed. I heard about him from Barkley. Reed was about speeding up via the ninety-second crown prep and increasing production. Reed was a smart guy, but there was something about him I didn't trust. He had a lot of good things to say, but mostly about speeding up and increasing production, but no mention of quality care. In the evening, some of us attending the seminar met in a Jacuzzi at the hotel. We shared stories. Bob Zabaknick was in that group. He was a consultant for the Professional Economic Bureau (PEB) in Minneapolis. He talked about his work with dentists. He talked about a Red Line, Blue Line, and Green Line to monitor expenses, savings, and profit. The Red Line was break-even, with no profit. The Blue Line was Red Line plus 10% profit. The Green Line was Red Line plus 20% profit. When he worked with dentists, once they got to the Blue Line, they quit. I found that fascinating, later on that subject. He suggested I meet Jim Trask, the President of PEB. So, I did. Trask's business was in Minneapolis. I drove to meet with him, and we met for a couple of hours. What he said made sense, and I began to work with Trask and his group.

Jim Trask was one of the smartest people I ever met. He knew more about the management of a dental practice than anyone I'd met before or since. He'd been a banker in North Dakota before he started the Professional Economic Bureau. He started PEB because he saw many dentists' accounting statements and realized they knew little about money and less about how to manage a practice. PEB had a database of more than 400 dental practices in the Midwest. Trask developed a management software program, the best I've ever seen. We were to record every procedure, canceled or changed appointment, every case presentation, every appointment, payment, and every recall appointment with a code on our daily pegboard sheet.

This was before in-office computers and before dental insurance had imposed its grip on dentistry. Each day, we would mail the daily sheet to PEB. A keypunch operator at PEB inputs the data into a main-frame computer. On the last day of the month, we sent in our expenses coded by categories. The next week, we got back a resource summary, which gave us an overview of the performance of every system in our practice. The resource summary gave me a complete picture of the performance of my practice. I still have an example of the Resource Summary Report.

The design of the PEB resource summary report taught me to look at the whole system and the key elements of our practice. I'm a big-picture person. I need to see the whole and then evaluate how the parts impact the whole. I worked with Jim Trask and PEB for ten years, from 1969-1978. With the PEB system, I could identify a weak system that was impacting the performance of my practice. We could also set goals for any system we wanted to improve. There were many benefits to this system, but most important, I knew what was going on in my practice. From 1969 to 1978, my practice grew 30% or more per year. Growth has its benefits and its problems. 30% is a very high increase in annual net profit. In 1978, our practice had gross revenues of $1.8 million with a 45% overhead. $1,800,000 is equal to $24,418,333 in 2024. That's inflation!

PEB's resource report evaluated the performance of:

- New Patient system

- Patient referral system

- Recall system

- Total treatment plans pending

- Total production by producer

- Accounts receivable

- Collections

- Expenses

- Credit extension and follow-up

- Financial Arrangement evaluation

- Down payment system

- Insurance system

- Appointment book control system

- Scheduling system

- Case Presentation system

- Patient planning and flow system

- Patient visits system—production per patient

- Radiology scheduling system

- Diagnostic system—how much dentistry was diagnosed per patient

  Expenses percentage budget system

- Administrative salaries as a percentage of collection

- Treatment salaries as a percentage of collection

- Hygiene salaries as a percentage of the collection

- Occupancy expense as a percentage of collection

- Front office expenses as a percentage of collection

- Equipment expenses as a percentage of collection

- Clinical supplies as a percentage of collection

Trask called this the *rule of sixes.'* Based on production. Below were the percentage goals.

- 6% for chairside salaries

- 6% for front office salaries

- 6% for hygiene salaries

- 6% for occupancy expense

- 6% for administrative supplies

- 6% for professional supplies

- 6% for equipment and furnishings

- 10% for laboratory expense

Trask's ideas about money aligned with Clason's laws of money. Jim taught me the Rule of Sixes and percentage budgeting. He said, "No matter how much you produce if you don't have a budget and stick with it, you won't be financially viable."

Jim Trask taught me to look at my practice as a complete system and a systems approach to management. I can't tell you how important that was. It gave me peace of mind. I gained deeper insight into how my practice worked. I understood what was working and what wasn't. I felt like I was in control. I learned why each system was important and how it impacted the performance of my whole practice. I spent several hours a week working on my practice with my team and my coach. I was learning a great deal and gaining confidence as well.

All this was contained in a two-page report. We had healthy performance criteria for each system. We could set goals for any system in our practice and track our results monthly.

Jim also taught me percentage budgeting with time. He taught the A—B—C idea of allocating time. A - time is the highest and best use of my time and talent. B - time is the time I spend preparing for A time and A procedures. C - time and C procedures reduce my effectiveness and should be stopped, delegated, or referred out.

I give Trask the credit of helping me produce more, and dramatically increase net profit with less stress and effort. It was through categorizing my procedures and time that I came to believe 'Less is More.' Percentage budgeting with money and time enabled me to work three days a week and earn more than I did working five days a week. I wanted to spend more time with my family, and I wanted to teach. Without the whole systems approach that I learned from Trask, I wouldn't have been able to work less, produce more, and have the time that I wanted in my life. The years with PEB taught me how to manage my dental practice effectively. I now had a foundation to build my practice and life on. I had control of money. I had control of time. I knew how to organize my practice and keep it organized as it grew. More on that later.

Although Trask didn't promote a three-day work schedule, his strategies enabled me to work three clinical days a week, work with people I enjoyed, do worthwhile work, and make a good income. My story is like others who refuse to give in and give up, refuse to live an ordinary life, refuse to be average, refuse the well-worn path of mediocrity, and refuse traditional disease care as the primary focus of their practice. We've all heard: "Seek and ye shall find!" "When the student is ready, the teacher appears." These sayings are true for me and for everyone. I learned that if I wanted something, and I wanted it bad enough, I'd find it.

Something else was happening. I was getting busier and busier. I felt like I was caught in the quality/quantity trap. I wanted to do quality, but I was too busy. I needed to slow down to do the quality of dentistry that satisfied me. Something was still missing. What was missing? I'd heard of Dr. LD Pankey. There was a lot of talk about Pankey at that time. I had the good fortune of saving a significant amount of money, but where would I put it so it would grow and I wouldn't lose it? I was making money, but not sure how to invest it so it would grow.

I heard Pankey was a wealthy dentist. Now, in my third year of practice, my wife and I would go to Florida to play tennis for a week. She loved tennis, and that was a way to get away, have fun, and spend fun time together. Two things bothered me. Something was missing in a case using the gnathology technique, and I needed to find a way to invest and keep what I was making. While on a tennis vacation in Florida, I called Dr. Pankey. There were no cell phones and no answering services in those days. Pankey answered the phone. I asked him several questions regarding the issues I was facing. The lack of definitive success with Gnathology, and how to invest the money I was making. We spoke for thirty minutes. He said, "Next week, Dr. Schuyler, Dr. John Anderson, and I are putting on a course in Ft. Lauderdale, and you need to be there."

Pankey told me it was going to be Clyde Schuyler's last public presentation. He also said he was going to do a Philosophy of Dentistry Course after that in the same hotel. What was I to do? I had another opportunity staring me in the face. I talked with my wife and suggested she fly home. I made the decision to stay in Florida and spend the next week taking the two seminars. I called Linda White, my secretary, and told her she was going to have to cancel my patients for the next week, and I told her why. Then, I called Dr. Pankey and signed up.

**What did I learn?**

Without Bob Barkley, Elliott Simon, and Jim Trask, I wouldn't be writing this today. Good ideas are one thing. Implementing good ideas was the key to my success. Looking back now, I realize Barkley gave me a purpose to practice dentistry. Barkley, Elliott Simon, and Jim Trask taught me how to do it. Without knowing how I couldn't have moved forward. The right people came into my life at the right time because I was looking for them. Allow me to repeat this: the right people will come into your life only when you look for them?

I had a purpose, guidelines for money and time, and a way to organize and manage my practice. Patients responded positively to my preventive approach to dentistry. Now, in my new office, I had a full schedule of putting out fires first and repairing the barn second. Our focus was prevention first. By that time, I was teaching at Iowa, and I was invited to join a small group of dentists studying Gnathology. In the first year, we completed a full case with the guidance and mentoring of Niles Guichet on a Denar D5A system. The next year, I completed two cases in the study club with Dr. Larry Huber, a prosthodontist and protege of Dr. Guichet.

Two cases worked well, and one didn't. Why didn't one work? At that time, the gnathological approach was missing something. My patient wasn't happy, and neither was I. The patient was the mother of a technician in Davenport, Iowa. I remember adjusting her goldwork several times after I seated her case. One morning, she was again in my office for an occlusal adjustment. While she was there, I had a phone call from her son, a dental technician in Davenport. These are his exact words. "I thought you knew what you were doing when I sent my mother to you." My response was, "I thought I knew what I was doing as well." I eventually ground through a couple of castings on several molars. Later, I redid the case when her TMJ was fully seated. Clearly, I had more to learn.

Later, I learned that two things were missing in Gnathology at that time. A verified centric relation before treatment and anterior guidance. Gnathology was based on how the joint moved, and the occlusion was built around various jaw movements that were recorded and input into an instrument. If the patient had acceptable anterior guidance and a verified centric relation, it worked. If a patient didn't have satisfactory anterior guidance and centric relation, the patient didn't do well. They had headaches, neck aches, and TMD pain.

Fast forward 31 years. I was invited to Dr. Tom Basta's training facility in San Francisco. Bio-Esthetics International was putting on a course in Basta's facility. I wasn't in the room for three minutes when Dr. Ron Roth, a renowned orthodontist, came up to me and said he wanted to talk to me. Roth was a pioneer in orthodontics done to a centric relation position. He took me into a small office and told me this story. The American Academy of Orthodontics has an annual meeting every year. Dr. Roth said he presented six completed cases showing the before and after models. He said many complimented him on his results. Then he said, "If they were so perfect, why did some patients end up with headaches?"

Then I told my story of grinding through some castings after I seated a case done with Gnathology. We both had come to a similar conclusion. Something had to be missing for our patients to have problems after the work was completed. Ron and I became close professional friends. We had similar experiences. Our patients weren't in a verified Centric Relation position. It seems like learning never ends. Later, Dr. Roth referred more than one hundred orthodontists to the Schuster Center. He said, "You can't practice what I teach without going through the Schuster Center."

# Chapter Five
# A Philosophy of Excellence and
# Professional Service

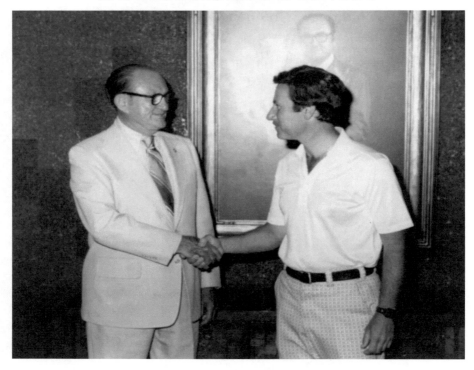

*Dr. LD Pankey (left) and Dr. Schuster*

*"I never saw a tooth walk into my office. . .The best interest of the patient should be the only interest of the dentist. . .Every person has one best treatment plan within them, and it's your job to go find it."*

*- Dr. LD Pankey*

The seminar with Pankey, Anderson, and Schuyler was another eye-opening experience. In the first seminar, Dr. Schuyler outlined the principle of anterior guidance and why it's essential to long-term stability in a person's natural dentition or dental rehabilitation. Drs. Pankey and Anderson outlined the Pankey-Mann-Schuylar technique with Dr. Schuyler.

The Philosophy of Dentistry seminar with Dr. Pankey was two and a half days. I felt like Dr. Pankey was speaking directly to me. I knew I'd found another great mentor for my practice and life. Dr. Pankey outlined a philosophy of life and dentistry. What he taught fit well with what I had been trying to do, but he gave me a much higher appreciation of what dentistry could do for people. It's difficult to describe the feeling. I knew I was in the right place. Pankey emphasized several things. He emphasized really getting to know each patient. He said, "You won't get to know a patient any better than you know yourself." He emphasized caring for the whole person, not just their teeth.

I'd been working to know myself and learn more about human behavior. Pankey put it together in a way that no one had done before or since. His philosophy was all inclusive of a dentist's life and practice. He said many times, "You take yourself wherever you go." My mother had said the same thing to me many times. I began to understand the importance of integrating my values into

59

my practice and life. Everything was beginning to make sense, to fit together. Reading <u>As A Man Thinketh</u> every day helped me understand how and why my thoughts directed my experience in practice and life. My mother said to me many times, "Life is like a deck of cards. It's not so much the cards you're dealt, but how you play them that makes the difference."

Dr. Pankey gave me a meaningful perspective, discussing both spiritual and financial rewards. I realized my initial distress in practice stemmed from a spiritual struggle, not just financial concerns. Pankey, who also focused beyond money, shared his transformation story. He had a similar early practice in rural New Castle, Kentucky, where removing teeth from uninformed patients devastated him, leading him to seek psychological help.

Barkley had a parallel experience. A high school cheerleader went elsewhere for dentistry and had all her teeth removed. Seeing her afterward deeply affected him. My early encounters with patients wanting teeth removed were similar, though I refused to extract healthy teeth. I struggled to connect and communicate with my patients, leading to physical and spiritual breakdowns. Hearing Pankey's story made me feel understood.

What I remember most about Dr. Pankey is that he emphasized the care of the whole person. He said things like this: *"I never saw a tooth walk into my office." "The best interest of the patient should be the only interest of the dentist." "Every person has one best treatment plan within them, and it's your job to go find it."*

Pankey taught me about people, about life, and about finding a better way to practice and live. He spoke about things my parents had spoken to me about. I remember him saying: *"Character is what you are. Reputation is what people think you are."* Pankey's philosophy of life and dentistry is timeless. I began to look at problems as opportunities to learn something, and my practice and life improved. Of all the teachers I've had in my life, Pankey impacted the quality of my life the most. I took eleven, yes eleven, Philosophy of Dentistry seminars with Dr. Pankey. I also took four with Dr. F. Harold Wirth, and several more with Loren Miller and John Anderson. I guess I'm a slow learner.

Sadly, most dentists are more interested in technique and technology than in people. Few dentists are interested in human development, communication, and relationships of depth. Pankey stressed the development of a significant relationship with each patient. He said it's important to know your patients' personalities, interests, what they do for a living, their family experience with dentistry, how they feel about themselves, and their general health and oral health status. He stressed the health of the whole person. He spoke a great deal about systemic health and its relationship to oral health. Further, he stressed the fact that I had to get my financial house in order so I could act in the patient's best interest and not my own. Then, in the first seminar, he quoted from the <u>Richest Man in Babylon</u> on numerous occasions. I knew I was going to use Dr. Pankey's philosophy as a model for my life and practice. Because of Dr. Pankey, I found my place in the world, and I fell in love with my profession.

As my vision became clear, my confidence and competence improved. I started the Pankey Continuum, which was four separate weeks. After the first session, I was hesitant to tell my wife that I had signed up for three more weeks. Every wife thinks their husband is already the best dentist in town. Dr. Pankey talked about a 'pyramid.' He said a large percentage of the population, maybe 50%, have a low dental appreciation and have little concern for oral health. The next higher group, 30%, has some concerns, and they can be educated to raise their Dental IQ, but will only go so far. Then, he said there are two higher groups (20%). Both groups of patients have high Dental IQ but have varying abilities to pay. He said many times, *"The cream rises to the top. In every town there are people willing and able to receive the best that you have to offer. There is no competition at the top because so few are willing to pay the price to get there."*

It was then that I decided to build a group practice. A practice that offered the finest level of dentistry possible, a practice created for patients who would choose health first and repair second. I bought a piece of property in Dubuque, Iowa, twenty-one miles from Dyersville. There was a house on the property and plenty of room to build a building with parking. My mother had seen the realtor sign on the property. She called me on a Tuesday and said, "*You've been talking about moving to Dubuque, and I see there is a lot for sale in a good location.*" One of the things Dr. Pankey stressed was, "*Get on a good corner. There are three things important in real estate: location, location, and location!*"

The next day, Wednesday, my afternoon off, I drove to Dubuque, looked at the property with a realtor, and put a deposit on it. Later, I wrote out a check to buy the property and the house for $55,000. I had to get the property rezoned. I went to every house in the neighborhood with a plan for my office. I promised them that the only way in or out of the parking lot would be on J.F. Kennedy Boulevard. The property was rezoned. I kept my promise. That was 1971! <u>My practice philosophy was formed.</u> The picture of the practice I wanted to create in Dubuque was clear in my mind. What I had learned from my mentors, Elliott Simon, Jim Trask, and Pankey, enabled me to bring my vision into reality. I built the building in 1972 and moved in late that year.

I spent 1972 with my team. We wrote and re-wrote a Mission statement until we agreed that it represented our thinking. I had it cast in bronze. Writing this statement and casting it was another defining experience in my professional life. This statement became the foundation for care delivered at Kennedy Dental Associates. People saw it when they entered our building. As you read this, you can sense the impact that Barkley had on my vision for dentistry.

LET IT BE KNOWN TO ALL WHO MAY ENTER....

THAT THIS BUILDING IS DEDICATED TO THE

PEOPLE IT SERVES. IT HAS BEEN DEDICATED

TO UPLIFTING MANKIND BY IMPROVING THE

HEALTH, APPEARANCE, AND WELL-BEING OF

PEOPLE. LET IT FURTHER BE KNOWN THAT

THE PEOPLE WHO WORK HEREIN HAVE

DEDICATED THEIR PROFESSIONAL LIVES TO

TREATING THE CAUSES OF DENTAL DISEASE,

RATHER THAN SIMPLY THE EFFECTS.

MICHAEL SCHUSTER 1973

In 1972, we built a 5400-square-foot building on two levels, two blocks away from the largest indoor shopping center in Iowa. I was in a good corner. I decided to limit my practice to periodontal therapy, occlusion, and reconstructive dentistry. Remember, I had completed a three-year part-time residency in Periodontics at the Iowa Dental School. I'd also completed two years and three full mouth cases with Niles Guichet over the previous two years. I was a busy boy. The only way I could limit my practice in Dubuque was to employ dentists as associates, leading to partners in different phases of dentistry. My first associate to become a partner was Dr. Bill Kuttler. His focus was endodontic therapy as well as general dentistry. Then Dr. Larry Donahue, whose focus was removable prosthetics and general dentistry. My good friend Dr. Wayne Moldenhauer, a Pediatric dentist, joined our practice as a partner the next year. We built out the lower level of the building so we had room for all of us.

Bobby Jungahan, from Davenport, asked to become my personal technician. He set up his lab in the basement of my house as our building was under construction in 1972. Later, two more technicians joined our practice as well. They all were doing my work. I can't say enough about the learning that occurred at that time. Working with my own technicians enabled me to produce the highest level of dental care possible. We used the best materials, and every case we did was a full wax-up. The wax-up served for both diagnosis and as the template of what we were planning. Every wax-up was approved by patients in writing before we began treatment. Patient demand increased, but we were determined to stay focused and centered on the outcomes we produced.

Don Allard, an orthodontist from Davenport, joined our practice on a part-time basis. His mandate was to do re-makes of former orthodontic cases. He was in our office one day the first year and three days every year after. In the second year Don was with us, he began treating children as well. He was so far ahead of his time. He wanted tonsils and adenoids out so that a child could breathe properly, which allowed the dental arches to grow properly. He also wanted third molars out before they were fully formed. I can't say how many third molars we removed, with minimum bone loss and complete healing. Allard did Phase I orthodontics earlier than most to ensure proper growth of the jaws and joints. Often, the kids didn't need Phase II orthodontics. It's amazing how much Don taught us all. He had been a gnathology technician, then a dentist, then an orthodontist. His knowledge and expertise added to the well-being of our patients.

Those were key learning years. With Bill, Larry, Wayne, Don Allard, and Jimmy Gertsema, we all worked together to develop a proper diagnosis for each person. Patients went through our Dental Fitness Program before repair treatment. Every patient had their joint stabilized before definitive restorative treatment. Every patient had a type-written Master Plan for prevention, diagnosis, prognosis, treatment agreed upon, and limitations of treatment. It was an amazing chapter in my life. Though it wasn't perfect, the people who worked with us at that time repeatedly said, "The time at Kennedy Dental Associates was the best professional experience in my career." Bill, Larry, Wayne, and Don Allard made wonderful contributions to the development of the practice.

**What did I learn?**

Working closely with my technicians transformed the quality of my dentistry. I handled every impression, trimmed every die, and mounted each case meticulously. This period, often called the golden age of dentistry, made me fall in love with every aspect of the field. Our primary focus was always on patient care, with the principle "Health is first" guiding us. Weekly team meetings reinforced our commitment to clinical excellence.

During this crucial period of my career, I learned from the best mentors, focusing on practical, hands-on experience. I developed "The Hour of Power," dedicating an hour each day to study and prepare, a habit I maintain. My evenings often involved working on cases, deepening my knowledge and skills. Accountability and feedback from mentors were essential in my growth.

Inspired by Maslow's studies on human behavior, I began to see the potential in each patient for higher health and wellness. I took full responsibility for my health, running five miles a day, and encouraged my patients to do the same. This holistic approach attracted like-minded patients and shaped my practice.

I rejected the sickness care model taught in dental school, aiming instead for excellence and a unique approach to dentistry. Barkley's influence and my early struggles pushed me to introspect and find answers within. I realized the need to understand patients' desires rather than assuming they wanted what I offered. This shift in perspective, aided by Maslow's "Motivation and Personality," revolutionized my practice and patient interactions.

**The most important thing I learned was that my perspective, my outlook, my attitude towards myself, and my patients had to change.** When I focused on changing myself, my whole world changed. I was busy telling patients what I thought they should do. When I started asking patients what they really wanted, I began to engage people. Began to connect with people. In my third year of practice, I was on a roll. I was moving forward. Patients were accepting not treatment, and me as well. I wanted my patients to respect me, to like me. The lack of acceptance and respect for me from my patients had been a key factor in the ulcer that I caused. I wanted to do worthwhile, meaningful work. I learned that good relationships with my team and patients were key to building the practice and life I had hoped for.

I was on the way, but someone else entered my life and changed it even more for the better: Dr. Charles M. Sorenson.

# Chapter Six
# The Power Shift

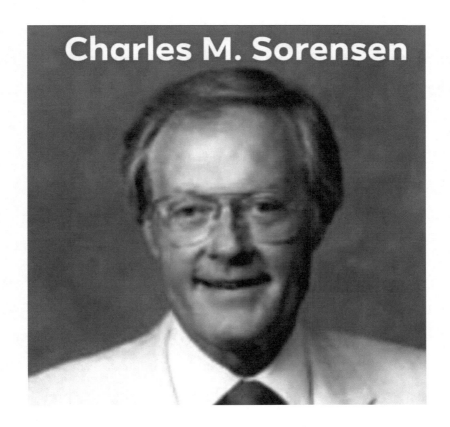

"Both the patient and the dentist create a transformative relationship. Both are changed for the better. Both get to keep their power. This type of relationship, though rare in our current culture, offers us hope for a better future."

*Dr. Charles Sorenson*

Dr. Pankey had a powerful impact on my life and practice. He gave me the idea of a group practice. But how was I going to form it? Thankfully, I had a close relationship with Jim Trask, and he recommended Dr. Charles Sorenson to help me engage the dentists and team members for the group practice. Charles was instrumental in helping me put together a humanistic team of people. Humanistic people have a higher concern for people than they do for things.

I employed Dr. Sorenson to help me with dentist and staff selection, but he taught me so much more. Several things need to be re-stated. Because of Robert Barkley, my focus on health first formed the purpose for my practice. Because of LD Pankey, I developed a more complete approach to listening to and caring for patients as individuals. Because of my training in periodontics and gnathology, I developed a practice that represented who I was and delivered a level of dentistry that had not been delivered previously in Eastern Iowa. At that time, as today, dentistry was pretty much a drill—fill—bill profession. There was only one other dentist in Iowa, Dr. Bill Brown, in Des Moines, who was a health-first dentist. We had instituted some significant alternative strategies in our practice, thanks to my early mentors.

I was becoming more effective, but I still had to learn another hard lesson. Barkley is given credit by some for Co-

Discovery, Co-Diagnosis, and Co-Development of treatment plans. He didn't share much of that with me. It was Charles Sorenson who gently flipped me on my head. Even though I was doing many things right, I was still trying to control the choices my patients made. This is difficult to describe. What initially put me in the hospital was a total lack of connection with my patients. I was busy trying to get my patients to do what I wanted them to do. I thought I was supposed to make the treatment plan and sell it to each patient.

Participative management was the rage in the early 70's. Maslow, Douglas McGregor of MIT, Carl Rogers, and others had developed a distinctly different theory of human Interaction and human motivation. McGregor's book, The Human Side of Enterprise, was vital to helping those who were interested in shifting the power of decision-making from the dentist to the patient. Over several years, Dr. Sorenson guided me in shifting the power of decision-making to the patient. This was not an easy time for me. There is stress in discovering a different way. I had to give up one way of thinking and go for a new, different way of thinking and behaving. Barkley and Pankey's influence showed me a way to practice and behave, but without Dr. Sorenson's help and guidance, I doubt I would have made the shift in thinking. Dr. Sorenson wrote an article called Power Shift! Power Shift is a profound statement of the shift in thinking that I experienced as a young dentist. (I've added the article by Dr. Sorensen in an appendix. I edited it with his permission some time ago.)

As a dentist, I can't let uninformed, uneducated patients make any choice they want. I'd be back in chaos. The key is to help patients make educated and informed choices. Most of what I had already created was helping people make informed choices. However, I did not completely let go of control over patients until I worked with Dr. Sorenson. It took time to make a shift in thinking of this magnitude. The idea that people are good and, when properly educated and informed, will make the best choices for themselves was dramatically different thinking. Previously, I doubted this was possible.

Helping people make good choices required that I slow down even more and spend even more time with patients.

1.  Listening to their dental story

2.  Sharing the Dreadful story. The Dreadful story was a vital key to changing the thinking of my patients.

3.  Showing pictures of health and disease and discussing both.

4.  Establishing the purpose for our relationship.

5.  Asking for permission to do a 'guided tour' of their mouth.

6.  Sharing three things that were core to my practice:

a. Worthwhile work.

b. Enjoyment, even fun in my practice.

c. Profit

7. Doing a comprehensive examination with the patient participating in every aspect of the examination.

8. Giving each patient a copy of Human Lifestyling.

9. Taking appropriate records.

10. Doing an 'initial review of findings' with the patient's photographs.

    a. Review of key points in Human Lifestyling.

    b. Establishing each patient's specific goals and the outcomes they wanted.

11. Having each patient go through an individually designed Dental Fitness program.

12. Doing a treatment discussion after the Dental Fitness program and/or Joint Stabilization.

The idea of a shared responsibility became increasingly important as I transitioned from my control over treatment planning and treatment choices to the patient's control to make good choices for themselves. It took time and dedication to principles. For some patients, this process was far easier than for others. Most patients have been conditioned to ask the doctor what should be done, relinquishing their power to choose for themselves. I'd say medicine and dentistry haven't changed much in the type of relationships that are formed. Dentists and physicians were in control until insurance began to determine what could and couldn't be done by restricting what treatment they would or would not pay for.

Thanks to Dr. Charles Sorenson, my thinking shifted even more, and my success rate increased to nearly 100%. I achieved what I wanted to achieve.

1. I wanted patients to take responsibility for their own health.

2. I wanted people to be free to make choices for themselves.

3. I wanted people to take responsibility for the outcomes of the choices they made.

4. I wanted people to keep all their teeth for their entire life.

5. I knew I couldn't do it alone. I knew I had to enroll people in caring for themselves.

The article, Power Shift, originally written by Dr. Charles Sorensen, confirmed what I had experienced. My early failure proved that the way I was thinking about people, their motivation, their involvement, and their decision-making process was flawed.

That's why I failed. I was trying to control people. I was trying to get patients to do what I thought they should do. I had fallen into the well-worn path of being an expert and making decisions for patients rather than with patients.

# Part Two

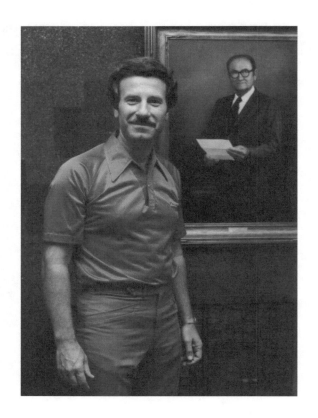

# How I Shared the Model and Created the First Business School for Dentists

*"We live in the shadow of giants."*

# Chapter Seven
# Teaching at the Pankey Institute
## The Birth of the Schuster Center

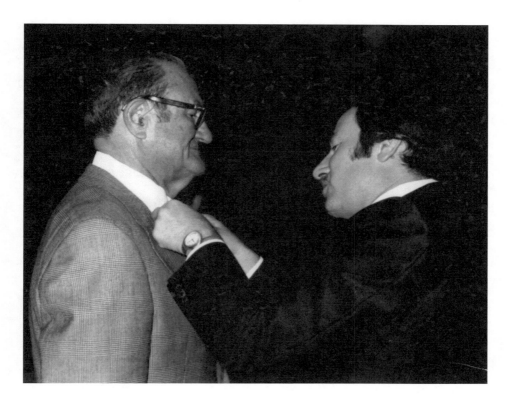

*Dr. LD Pankey and Dr. Mike Schuster adjusting Pankey's tie.*

*"Mike, you've got to keep teaching this. The dentists need to hear from someone who is doing it!"*

*Dr. LD Pankey*

I finished the Pankey Continuums in 1973. In my last Continuum week, Dr. Loren Miller, the Director of the Pankey Institute, asked me if I would like to be a Cadre (core faculty) at the Institute. He explained that I would have a teaching commitment for two weeks a year and become part of a group that would get together several times a year for more intensive learning. I said yes to this opportunity. Being involved as a Cadre at Pankey was another defining opportunity that ultimately changed the course of my life. Because of various circumstances on the part of other Cadre members (there were fifteen of us), I ended up teaching more than one week a month for twelve years. That was more than 144 weeks of teaching, studying, learning, and sharing with colleagues at the Pankey Institute. I was teaching them, but our students were teaching me as well.

When on assignment, I'd go for walks and runs with participants. We had many lunches, dinners, and late-night discussions. Because I could wax and cast, I became a primary teaching Cadre in Continuum III. In this course, students prepped teeth on manikins, took impressions, poured models, waxed up a quadrant, and then the faculty cast the wax up in technique metal. This was to be a true test of what was learned in the first two sessions. The technicians and I would stay up late at night, burning out the wax patterns and casting onlays for the next day. I taught all four courses but primarily taught Continuum III and IV.

I was fortunate to teach many weeks with Henry Tanner, who many considered to be one of the finest restorative dentists who ever lived. Working side-by-side with Dr. Tanner brought us closer together. Henry taught me to involve students in learning. He taught by the Socratic Method. He believed the answer to questions and problems lies within the student. The teacher's role is to help the student discover the answer. Henry and I taught quite a few seminars together in various cities in the US. It was a great learning experience with Dr. Tanner. He continued to teach in various study clubs throughout the US after he was let go by Chris Sager, the Director of the Pankey Institute.

What I learned from the students changed my perspective regarding dentists and dentistry. Outside the classroom, most of the conversations weren't about dentistry but about the various problems the dentists were facing. They had tax problems, not enough profit problems, lack of time for family problems, staff problems, and saving money problems.

The most common recurring problem the students complained about was that they couldn't get patients to move forward with comprehensive care that we were teaching at the Institute. Over and over, the same problems persisted: people problems, staff problems, lack of time problems, patient acceptance of treatment problems, tax problems, and money problems, all leading to high levels of stress. The internal conflicts they were experiencing prevented them from doing the level of dentistry we were teaching. The most common complaints I heard were, "You can't do comprehensive dentistry in my town!" and, "The people in my area don't have money or time for Pankey-style dentistry!"

It didn't take long to realize that dentists coming to the Pankey Institute were experiencing problems similar to those I had in my first year in practice. The stress that made me sick was like what our students at the Pankey Institute were experiencing. Just like when I started in practice, they had no purpose, no stated philosophy of practice, no management method, no money or time strategies, and ineffective new patient processes. Everything then, as today, was about going faster, doing piecework, and meeting money goals. They hadn't learned how to help patients make good decisions. Dentists believed then, as now, that their problems would be solved if they learned more technical dentistry. They were lost, just as I had been.

One of my assignments, as a Cadre, was to get the class together in the evening and go over the key steps and strategies they could implement when they went back to their practices. Because of my personality, I told it as I saw it. One evening, when the class was being dismissed after several hours of discussions, Dr. Pankey was waiting for me as I walked out. Each room at the Institute had a microphone wired into Dr. Pankey's office. Dr. Pankey had been listening to my talk from his office. As I walked out, he said, "You've got to keep doing this. They need to hear from someone who is doing it!" That was the beginning of a deeper relationship I developed with Dr. Pankey. After that, we spoke frequently and often had lunch together.

My practice had evolved quickly because of the many wonderful people that came into my life and because I was willing to do the work necessary to build the practice I wanted. My practice became a model practice for the Pankey Philosophy. Part of our Cadre assignment was to welcome other Pankey students into our practices to observe. Over the next several years, at least once a month, we had dentists and team members observing our practice. On many weekends, couples would come to Dubuque, and my wife and I would help them find balance in their lives.

I taught at the Pankey Institute one week a month. I worked twelve clinical days a month, and the other dentists worked in our practice while I was away teaching. Between my practice, teaching at the Pankey Institute, hosting dentists in the office, and counseling couples, all the activities were overtaking our lives!

**The Schuster Center is born**.

Lives change when beliefs change. Each of you has your own beliefs. A simple explanation is that each of us has a 'belief window' through which we see, read, and hear everything.

We filter all information through our 'belief window.' If we agree with it, we see it, but if we don't agree, new ideas don't get through. Beliefs can change, and if your beliefs change, your behavior will as well. Life is a full-time school of lessons. You either learn the lessons and change your behavior, or the lessons are repeated throughout your life.

Students of the Schuster Center have experienced many shifts in thinking. Not every student experienced all of these changes in thinking and behavior, but many did.

These shifts in thinking created transformations in their lives. Below are a few:

- **From production-centered to profit-centered.**

- **From money-centered to patient-centered.**

- **From repair/disease focus to health focus.**

- **From more is more to less is more.**

- **From transactional relationships to transformational relationships.**

- **From five clinical days a week to three clinical days a week.**

- **From two weeks off to eight weeks off.**

I made a life-changing decision. From my firsthand experience teaching and interacting with students at Pankey, I understood dentists had a tremendous need for help. I decided to create a place where dentists could come and learn, resolve their problems, create the practice they wanted, and implement what we were teaching at the Pankey Institute: comprehensive, whole-person dentistry. Because of my beliefs, I knew it had to be a health-first style of practice. The vision of the <u>Center for Professional Development</u> was formed. (Later renamed the Schuster Center.) With a picture in my mind, the idea of a Business School had formed.

I remember like it was yesterday (in 1975), cornering LD Pankey in the hallway and stepping into a room together. Dr. Pankey didn't like to be cornered. I told him about the problems students expressed to me. I related that I wanted to create a place where dentists could learn how to implement what we were teaching at the Pankey Institute. I didn't yet have a complete picture of the curriculum, where it would be, and how I would pull it off. I just knew that I was called to do it. I also knew it couldn't be done in Dubuque, Iowa.

It took three years to convince my wife to support the idea. Each year, she would say NO to the prospect of moving, starting over, and building the Center. In 1975, I wrote out the Mission of the Schuster Center. It reads:

*"We believe that every individual has Infinite Worth and unlimited*

*potential for growth, and when given correct information,*

*combined with the right support, any worthwhile purpose can be*

*accomplished.*

*We are dedicated to improvement, innovation, integrity, and*

*excellence in everything that we do.*

*Our mission is to nurture the spirit of every individual we touch,*

*and to empower people and organizations to*

*significantly increase their performance capability in*

*order to achieve worthwhile purposes through learning, living,*

*and teaching sound principles of life and business.*

*The Center Team*

I met with two different groups to go over our financial position. I asked them, "Are we prepared financially to make a move, start a new practice, and create the Schuster Center?" After their analysis, both groups told us that we were in a financial position to do it. It was now late 1977. My wife and I attended a retreat with Dr. F. Harold Wirth in New Orleans, as well as other Cadre members and their spouses. The name of the retreat was "Never Cease to Love." Another wonderful experience with my friend Harold Wirth. We then flew to Arizona, where we attended a timely retreat with Avrom King, which was "Value Clarification, Conflict Resolution, and Goal Setting." This was exactly where we were in our lives. We reviewed our values individually and together. We identified the conflicts that were interfering with a life choice that I hoped we could make together. Then, together, we set our goals.

These two retreats helped us define what we wanted, why we wanted it, and when and where to begin it. My wife JoAnn still had considerable resistance. Why should we leave the ideal situation we had built? We were, by all measurements, on top of our profession. We had a great practice, friends, a community we enjoyed, and a wonderful lifestyle. Saving and investing money, we had accumulated more than $2.75 million dollars in 10 years! I never could have done this without the wonderful people that came into my life. I couldn't blame her for resisting leaving Iowa. However, the call to create this place, which we called the Center for Professional Development, was stronger. My purpose and what I do with my life have always been more important than money. Money makes things possible, but we still have to make the commitment to do it.

During the retreat with Avrom King, we went for a drive in North Scottsdale. We went out Scottsdale Road and turned east on Pinnacle Peak. The last two miles weren't paved yet, and we drove up into the foothills of the McDowell Mountains. At the end of a cul-de-sac was a five-acre lot that looked over the entire valley of Phoenix. The sun was setting as we got out of the car and walked part of a lot that was for sale. I remember turning to JoAnne and asking her,

"Can you see yourself here?" With tears in her eyes, she said, "Yes". The next day, I met with the owner/broker and made an offer on the property. The builder/owner was Greg Hancock. Before we left Arizona, our offer was accepted. The start of our new home and the Center for Professional Development was underway.

I knew that I had the information, the knowledge, and the process that had changed my life for the better. I had worked with a study club in Minneapolis/St. Paul on referral from Jim Trask. The members of the study dramatically improved the quality of their practices as I helped them implement the principles and strategies I had learned about money, time, organization, and the new patient process. I worked for two years with this group, 1973-1974.

A method to build a comprehensive, health-focused, person-centered practice and life was born. Was I just to use it for myself, or should it be shared? I choose to share it. The next most important part was to organize a teaching process where dentists could learn, grow, and thrive. Anything that is worthwhile should be shared. Since I already knew firsthand that it worked, I re-evaluated how I had done it, and that formed the foundation of the step-by-step curriculum that I created at the Schuster Center. We call this method of practice the Schuster Model.

# Chapter Eight
# The Schuster Model for Practice Success

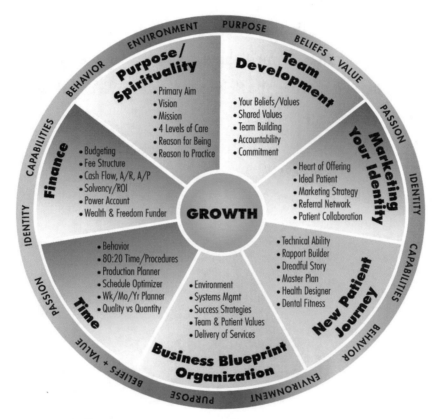

## The Growth Matrix™

*"What you are is God's gift to you, and what you do with it is your gift to God."*

*Mary Schuster*

In chapters 1-7, I shared what I had discovered. It wasn't my intention to create a new model of professional practice. My goal was to make my life work. As I look back at my life experience, I see that I was born into a family of seekers and teachers. I was a restless child, but once I found a purpose for my life, there was no stopping my progress. Every time I experienced a major problem, I sought help, and each time, I found the person, the idea, and the strategy that I needed to advance.

Many people impacted my life. Some I knew personally, including my mother and father, Mary Ellen and Edward, Robert Barkley, and LD Pankey, Jim Trask. Some I never met, like Abraham Maslow. There were many others who guided me, assisted me, and taught me the principles and strategies that helped me express my potential. One thing is extremely important. We are all offered opportunities. If you don't take advantage of opportunities, you get stuck. People don't see opportunities because they aren't looking for them. In other cases, people don't believe they deserve to be happy, content, or fulfilled.

***Seek, and you shall find! But you must seek!!***

As humans, we all have potential unless there is some mental or physical disability or addiction that thwarts it. She would say that what we all want is happiness, peace, and contentment. How we arrive at that may be different, as there is no single path. Yet, when

I first began my practice, I was miserable. I was suffering. When a person suffers emotionally, the body usually experiences the effect of the suffering. The body doesn't lie!

I worked hard in high school, college, dental school, and two years in the US Navy. I took many technical courses while in the Navy and even taught part-time at Temple Dental School. Yet, I wasn't prepared for what I experienced in private practice. So, this book, and what I am sharing with you, is about what I discovered and put into practice to change the experience and course of my life. The major discoveries occurred in the first five years of practice. In my fourth full year in practice, I went through the Pankey Institute's program.

I didn't know that accepting the teaching opportunity at the Pankey Institute would change the direction of my life. Dentists were coming to the Institute to learn technical dentistry. However, at breakfast meetings, dinners, walks, and runs together, they complained about the same things I had complained about—money problems, tax problems, savings problems, time problems, patients rejecting comprehensive treatment problems, staff problems, not enough patients, too many patients, self-esteem, and self-confidence problems.

The majority were suffering from the same problems I had suffered just five years before! As I look back, I've asked myself many times why I was so blessed to have wonderful people enter my life at such an early age and in the order that they appeared. Was it blind luck? Was I just in the right place at the right time? Was it synchronicity? Or was I being prepared to serve others as well as myself? I discovered in five years what no one discovered in a lifetime of practice. Why me? I believe I was called to help dentists in a profound way.

I believe I was called. I was called to create a school where dentists could discover, learn, and develop. The school would enhance their knowledge, self-esteem, and self-confidence. I presented the idea of the school I wanted to create to Dr. Pankey in 1975, and he was all in. He said the school I was planning was sorely needed in dentistry. With Pankey's blessing, I was determined to create the first business school in dentistry. I named it the Center for Professional Development. Today, it is called the Schuster Center. No one can really learn and develop without being a student in a school. There are many kinds of schools. The type of school that really develops students has certain characteristics.

*Dr. Schuster, Keynote speaker at the Hinman meeting*

**What constitutes a true school?**

We think we know what a school is, but most of what we call schools are not schools in the true sense. So, what constitutes a school? A traditional school teaches classes that, in most instances,

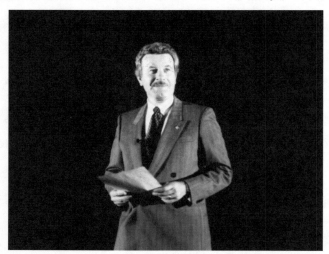

don't relate to each other. You take a class in Math, and fifty minutes later, the bell rings, and you go to the next class in English. On and on! The classes don't relate to each other or support each other. We learn to study for a test and move on. There is little or no learning. I wanted to create a different kind of school. A school that taught key principles and strategies for a specific outcome, which was defined by each student.

I wanted to create a school where dentists could learn the principles, the methods, and the strategies to create the practice and life they wanted. I wanted them to be profitable and to have a plan to create wealth (abundance.) I wanted dentists to gain control of the forces that dominate most lives, money, and time and learn to create meaningful, worthwhile relationships with everyone in their sphere of influence. I wanted them to be happy, satisfied, and fulfilled. I wanted to help dentists conquer their frustration and, often, their anger at the environment around them.

These are the characteristics of a school.

1st: A school is a place you go to learn something. Learning requires doing, not just listening or seeing, but acting on what you are taught.

2nd: A real school requires a 'practice field' or a place to test and implement the concepts and strategies presented.

3rd: Each person learns and implements at a different rate. Therefore, each person must have a personal tutor, guide, or coach.

4th: Any person who teaches or coaches at the school must first understand the principles and concepts being taught and have implemented them in their life and practice themselves. A true school must have a faculty who 'walk their talk.'

5$^{th}$:    Learning requires four elements:

A.  A goal, end result, or purpose to learn (WHY.)

B.  An idea, concept, or theory must be taught (WHAT.)

C.  That idea or concept must be converted into a strategy (The HOW.)

D.  The student must act on the strategy (HOW.)

E.  As the student acts, feedback and accountability are required for learning.

I knew this because it's the way I learned. It's the way everyone learns. I learned from those who both taught and implemented what they were teaching. Barkley walked his talk. He taught me what he had been doing in his own practice. Pankey taught me, but he taught me what he had done in his practice and his life. My parents taught me, but they also lived according to what they taught me. As adults, we learn by doing, by practicing, and by getting feedback.

I knew this worked. I began to think of my practice as a school, a place where my patients could come to learn something. In fact, I was determined that each patient would learn something at every appointment. I found that as my patients learned more about the cause of dental disease, they took a more active role in preventing disease.

*"If a person doesn't take responsibility for their decision, they won't take responsibility for the outcome."*

The more I learned about something, the more interested and competent I became. Understanding money improved my ability to make, keep, and invest it. Learning about time and organization enhanced my efficiency, while mastering relationship-building improved my interactions at home, with my team, and with patients.

I applied these learning principles to create a school within my practice and later founded the Center for Professional Development for dentists. Maslow's theory taught me that unmet basic needs lead to distress, and fulfilling these needs brings well-being. Maslow gave me hope and a model for personal growth, even if he didn't show me the exact path.

Forming a philosophy and purpose for my practice came first, inspired by Barkley. Upset by high taxes in my first year, I sought financial control and was guided by Elliott Simon to read *The Richest Man in Babylon*. Time control and organization came next with Jim Trask, who taught me to feel in control of my practice.

Dr. Charles Sorenson helped me develop meaningful, trusting relationships with patients. Studying with Carl Rogers and

William Glasser further refined my approach. The practice model I developed mirrors Maslow's: survival first, then safety and security, followed by relationships. Gaining control over money and time boosted my confidence, organizing my practice around my purpose made it truly mine, and building deeper relationships reduced stress and enhanced my practice.

Today, I'm retired from a practice I loved. I learned to love dentistry because I love making a big difference in people's lives, and I love crafting things with my hands. Dentistry became a personal expression of the person I wanted to be. Establishing trusting relationships is essential for comprehensive, whole-person dentistry.

The shift from 'transactional relationships' to 'transformational relationships' took time, study, practice, and feedback. Transformational relationships can only be learned from someone who has created them. Transformational relationships are significantly different from transactional relationships. Creating transformational relationships is a process by which a patient's thinking changes and then behavior changes. Behavior doesn't change unless a person's mind changes. I knew I wanted to make a big difference in the lives of my patients. To do this, I had to learn how to establish deeper, more meaningful, trusting relationships. The theory of creating transformational relationships is a vast but simple process. A traditional process of helping is when a dentist sells solutions that he knows how to do or decides for the patient what should be done. A different relationship is when the dentist helps the patient discover the causes of disease and engages each person in an educational discovery process. Over time, and the amount of time varies with each patient, the patient becomes free to make the best choice for themselves.

You don't need a relationship to treat someone's disease, but you do need a significant relationship to help a person become healthy.

I taught and coached in my school for forty years, from 1978-2018. What I learned in those forty years is what we hope to pass on to you in this book. This book is not a school, but hopefully, it may show you a path, a road you may want to travel. We are all, as we live our lives, writing our own stories. Our stories will have ups and downs, successes and failures. But I hope, at some point, you will look back at your life and say,

*"I did it my way and with the help of those who lived before because of their wisdom and guidance. I am happy and satisfied with my life."*

The day I learned to put my patients' well-being first was the day my life was transformed. It is in the giving that we receive. I can honestly say, "The more I gave, the greater value I created for each person I served, the more I received."

# Chapter Nine
# The Power of Purpose

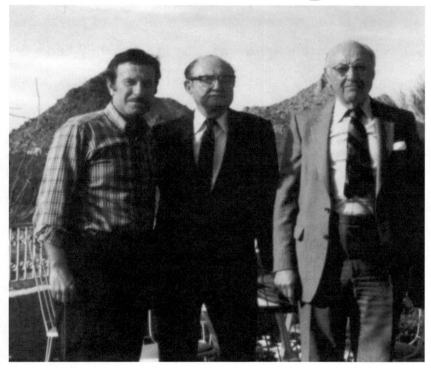

*Dr. Mike Schuster, Dr. LD Pankey, and Dr. Harold Wirth*

*"The two most important days of your life are:*

*The day you were born. The day you found out why."*

*Mark Twain*

Many dentists have a good life, but they sense that something is missing. They don't feel quite right but don't know why. We each develop a pattern of living. That pattern works, or it doesn't. Early in life, we are under the influence of parents, family, and teachers. Most attempt to mold us to what they believe is the right pattern of living, the pattern they have lived or hope to have lived. To live whole and complete lives, we must find our own way and develop our own pattern of living. Little is done to help us discover our gifts and our strengths. Nothing is done to help us discover our purpose. The school does nothing to help us discover who we really are, what our naturally motivated gifts are, and how to develop them and use them. I never had a class or course on discovering my natural gifts or on how or why to discover purpose.

I discovered my professional purpose in my second year of practice. It changed my practice and life in profound ways. I related this in an earlier chapter, but it's worth repeating. I was fortunate to have an early health crisis that forced me to ask myself why I was in practice in the first place.

At first, my practice was mostly about me and what I wanted. Also, I wanted to make a difference for my patients, but I had no idea how to do it. I had no clue about what my patients really wanted. I wrote earlier that Dr. Bob Barkley took me under his wing and helped me think in a different way.

In the hospital for a week, I began to ask myself questions I never had before. What do my patients really want? Why did patients resist what I offered them? What were they telling me they really wanted? I came up with these responses:

1.  My patients wanted no dentistry or as little as possible.

2.  They wanted to spend as little money on their teeth as possible.

3.  They wanted to be free from pain, discomfort, sensitive teeth, and head and neck pain.

Many in the small rural town where I worked thought that if they got all their teeth out, their problems would be over.

I read a book by Benjamin Franklin, in which he wrote out his 13 values. His book inspired me to write out what I believed about dentistry, and I wrote out my 13 beliefs:

1.  I believe decay and gum disease are the most common yet most preventable diseases known to mankind.

2.  I believe that decay and gum disease are controllable but not curable.

3.  I believe people want to be free from the pain and discomfort of gum disease.

4. I believe people want to be free from the pain and discomfort of decay and sensitive teeth.

5. I believe people want to be free from facial pain and headaches associated with decay, gum disease, and malocclusion.

6. I believe all patients deserve to be educated in a non-threatening environment relative to the causes, prevention, and treatment of these primary diseases: gum disease, decay, and malocclusion.

7. I believe all patients should be offered preventive and treatment choices that are consistent with their needs, wants, and values.

8. I don't believe in manipulating or struggling with patients to get them to do something they should want for themselves.

9. I won't care more for the teeth and health of any patient than they care for themselves.

10. I won't rescue patients. I'll provide options and opportunities for them to choose the level of care that is consistent with their values.

11. I believe all people have the right to choose health, but I also believe that people have the right to suffer from pain and disease.

12. I believe that people who choose health want a complete and thorough examination and a thorough Master Plan for present and future health. I believe it is my moral obligation to provide this for every patient I have the privilege to serve.

13. I believe all patients should have an education appointment to completely educate them on the causes and crippling effects of dental disease.

Thinking about each of my core beliefs helped me discover my practice purpose. What if I were to focus my practice on helping people get exactly what they told me they wanted? Not necessarily what they were telling me, but what deep, inside, they really wanted. Discovering my purpose changed my outlook regarding my patients and profession.

- What if I could help people become pain-free, disease-free, and healthy?

- What if I could help people spend as little money on their teeth as possible?

- What if I could help people have as little dentistry done in their lifetime as possible?

- What if I could help them eliminate discomfort, pain, and constant repair?

- What if I could help people keep all their teeth for life?

I went over and over these questions and came up with a statement of Practice Purpose that changed everything in my practice.

*"My purpose is to help you keep all your teeth for life."*

My purpose:

- Influenced how I spoke to people.

- Gave me positive energy and a new vision for my practice.

- Changed the focus of my practice.

- Changed how I organized my practice.

- Changed how I introduced patients into my practice.

- Changed how I organized treatment plans. I helped patients control the disease before repair.

- Gave me a definite focus for my practice.

- Enabled me to share my purpose with every patient in my practice.

- Inspired both my team and me with a reason for everything we did.

- Separated my practice from traditional, repair-oriented dentists.

- Was the best marketing strategy I could have created.

- Gave me an identity in the community.

I would not have discovered my purpose without the influence of Dr. Robert Barkley. Everything, then and since, has been influenced by my purpose. The orientation, focus, and structure of my practice changed dramatically. My practice took off.

Before, I felt disconnected from my patients. I resented the very people I was working for. I literally hated going to work. Sunday before every Monday, I'd get sick to my stomach because I knew I wasn't going to have a good day. I call it "Sunday sickness." Anyone who has enough of these days is going to get sick, as I did!

My purpose was everywhere: in my welcome letters to patients, on my practice brochure, and in every written review of findings for each patient. With a new energy and a new vision for my practice, I shared my purpose in words, in writing, and in action.

My practice purpose developed from my life purpose. I knew I wanted to make a difference in people's lives. I initially found myself trapped in a reactive mode. I felt trapped and didn't have a clear picture in my head or the words to communicate it. I wanted to help people, not watch them destroy their health over time.

Writing this book has forced me to look back at my life. When my practice wasn't going well, my life wasn't going well either. Further, my practice suffered when my personal life wasn't in harmony with my values. I found it impossible to disconnect my practice life from my personal life.

I met hundreds of dentists while teaching at the Pankey Institute, the Dawson Center, LSU Cosmetic Continuum, Bio-Esthetics International, and the Schuster Center for Professional Development. Purpose is the most common missing element in nearly every dental practice I've encountered. You are a system composed of elements that work together to enable you to live. If any one of your critical organs is weakened, your whole body is weakened. Your practice is a system, and each element is critical to the overall performance of your practice. If any critical element of the seven that I discovered is weak, then your practice will be weak. Each element impacts the performance of every other element. Let's review the Model I created:

1. **Money**

2. **Time**

3. **Organization**

4. **Sales/Communication**

5. **Marketing**

6. **People**

7. **Purpose**

I bet you know that Money (1) is critical to surviving and thriving. Time (2) is a critical element; time is how you spend your life! Most dentists have little appreciation for Organization (3) and usually abdicate organization to a consultant! Most dentists have little interest in Communication/Sales (4) but do have an interest in Marketing (5). People/Team (6) are not normally a priority. Purpose (7) is often assumed but rarely evident or clarified.

Purpose is invisible, and it gets the least attention. Money problems are visible. You know when you run out of money before the end of the month. You know when your payables are growing. You know when your revenues are declining. You know if you have money in your account at the end of the month or not. Time is another one of those invisible elements. We quantify time with minutes, hours, days, weeks, and months, but time itself is invisible.

Ask any 70-year-old about time, and they will say, *"I don't know where the years went."* The older you are, the faster time goes! That's relativity, according to Einstein.

Some elements are measurable, and others are not so much. Each element affects the performance of every other element and impacts your whole practice system, the same way each organ, heart, lungs, liver, and kidney, impacts your body's health. If any element is weak, it will impact the performance of every other element and your entire practice system. So, what is the purpose?

- It's your primary aim.

- It's why you do what you do.

- It's your reason for being.

- It's your reason for being in practice.

- It's your Identity.

- It's your inspiration, what gets you up and gets you going every day.

- Purpose is why you were born.

I believe each of us is born with gifts and a purpose. However, your gifts and your purpose must be discovered. Every person has a reason to be here. Purpose is the reason you were born.

From birth to death, each of us is on a silent quest to discover our purpose. Many never do. You can make a living without a defined purpose, but you won't be inspired. You won't love what you do, nor will you be fulfilled. Purpose gives direction to your life. Purpose defines what you do with your life.

People don't focus on purpose because they don't appreciate its importance. When I discovered my purpose, I began to feel alive, complete, and in harmony with myself and others. Had I not discovered my purpose in practice, I would have quit dentistry.

Purpose is evasive because many people are dominated by money and things, whether they admit it or not. Money and things can never fill the void of a lack of purpose and meaning. I never let money dominate my life. Purpose defines you and what you do with your time and talent.

My purpose wasn't about me but about my patients. My thirteen beliefs weren't about me but how I could transform the lives of my patients. It motivated me to find more and more ways to help my patients become disease-free and healthy. It inspired the people I worked with. We developed a shared purpose. Our purpose was so important that we engraved it on a bronze plaque. People saw it when they entered our building. It was also in calligraphy in several areas of the office. It was on every written review of findings and in every initial letter we sent to our patients. We talked about our purpose every morning at the staff round. We opened team meetings with a statement of purpose: why we are here and why we do what we do.

Every relationship of any importance must have a purpose. Without a purpose, you have no direction or rudder and will more than likely focus on yourself and how much money you are making. Money is no substitute for purpose. If you put money before purpose, you're in for a long, difficult, unfulfilled life. You may make plenty of money, but you won't be fulfilled.

Every business has two missions: an Economic Mission and a Service Mission. Unfortunately, most dentists and consultants put the Economic Mission first and rarely, if ever, think about the Service Mission. I know the model I created goes against traditional thinking. That is precisely why it is A Better Way to Practice. Most dentists have adopted the wrong model. The secular model puts your needs, goals, and wants ahead of your patient's needs, wants, and goals. It works up to a point, and then it doesn't. No one can fill the void of purpose and meaning in life with money and things. No one. The psychologist's offices are filled with people without a defined purpose, a reason to exist. They have stuff but always need more stuff because they aren't fulfilled or at peace with themselves.

Meeting LD Pankey was a defining time in my life. I was thirty-one. I completed the Pankey Continuum when I was thirty-three. Dr. Loren Miller, the director of the Pankey Institute, invited me to be a teaching Cadre at the Pankey Institute. I said yes to the opportunity. While teaching at the Institute, I took many walks and had many runs, breakfasts, and dinners with students. Most dentists were coming to the Institute for technical training. However, our conversations were about problems of:

- Not enough money.

- Paying too much in taxes.

- Complaining about employees and their lack of commitment.

- Working too hard.

- Not having enough time for fun and recreation.

- Feeling a lot of pressure and stress.

- Couldn't get patients to accept comprehensive treatment.

- In spite of a lot of technical CE, they were still doing piecework dentistry.

- Feeling pressures of insurance limitations.

- Believed they couldn't do Pankey comprehensive dentistry in their town.

These were many of the same problems I had experienced! I learned about their problems because they felt free to talk about them. They believed that because they were out of town, whatever they said wouldn't get back to those in their community. This pattern repeated itself over and over. Clearly, these weren't average dentists, yet they were stuck. They were so busy trying to solve their own problems that they didn't have the time or energy to focus on the problems their patients were facing.

A second professional purpose was born within me. Something instilled in me by my parents was to use the gifts and knowledge I gained to help others. I want to make a significant difference in the lives of the people I serve. The lack of this core need made me sick in the first eighteen months of my practice. Once I began to make a significant difference in the lives of my patients, my life and my health changed for the better.

As I witnessed the pain, the frustration, and the emotional and spiritual pain the dentists at the Pankey Institute were experiencing, I began to think about how I could help them. Perhaps what I had learned could transform their lives as mine had. After two years of teaching at the Pankey Institute, one week every month, I told Dr. Pankey that "I want to create a place where dentists can find themselves." Those were my exact words. Dr. Pankey said, "You must do it. Dentists need this so much."

I wouldn't have had the life I've had without the guidance of Drs. Barkley and Pankey. There are others, but these two dentists inspired a purpose within me that I never would have discovered on my own. The gifts you and I were born with must be discovered and developed. It will be your purpose that will inspire you to develop your gifts. My core purpose has never changed. **My life purpose is to transform lives**. I found a way to do this in my practice by helping people become healthy and disease-free. Over fifty years, my purpose in practice has never changed. I also found a way to transform the lives of dentists. It's the practice development method that I discovered and described in this book, A Better Way to Practice Dentistry.

In 1979, our first year in Arizona, I wrote a book which outlined the model I created,

Developing a Dental Practice for Excellence. It was later translated into Japanese by Quintessence. I lectured several times a month for thirty-five years all over the United States, Canada, and Puerto Rico. We started giving retreats in our home in Pinnacle Peak and established our school. From 1978 to 2018, we graduated nearly 4,000 dentists from our school in Arizona. Over that time, I wrote and published more than twenty programs, manuals, and books. I traveled more than ten million miles in that time. Speaking to study groups, national meetings, seminars, and workshops, we scheduled ourselves. I coined the <u>Profit-Ability Management Method</u> in 1983 and did many seminars with that title. More than 100,000 dentists bought tape and video programs and attended seminars. I lectured for more than 1,000 days and continue to do so today.

We established advanced programs for our graduates: Mastery, Leadership, and CEO. In 2006, together with a group of twenty key alumni, we created a new program, Performance Coach, which remains active today. The Performance Coach was created so that dentists could continue their mental, emotional, financial, and spiritual development. What I learned on the speaking tour motivated me to write <u>The Science of Creating Wealth.</u>

Over the years, we have partnered with Stephen Covey, Robert Fritz, Jacob Needleman, and James Hollis. Each became personal friends as well as professional colleagues. They added insights and positive energy to our cause. They believed in the principles and the methods by which we enabled dentists to live an extraordinary life and practice.

As I write this, I'm in the process of forming a study club based on the theme of this book. I want to continue to share the good news of the Principles, Strategies, and methods we've discovered in our journey. If you want a better practice and a better life, this is one way, perhaps not the only way, to create it. In the beginning and the end, what you do with your life is in your head, hands, and heart.

If you walk your talk, live what's in your heart, stand up for your beliefs, put your money where your mouth is, follow through on your promises, and do what you say you will do—your practice will thrive. You'll be more trusted, more powerful, and more successful in every arena of your life. You'll have more committed staff and be content and at peace with yourself.

It is a privilege to share this with you. It was Dr. Tim Leary's idea to write this book. Dr. Leary is an exceptional person who happens to be a dentist, a friend, and an advocate of the method that transformed his life and hundreds of others. This book was written to share good news, to share a process and theory that has proven to work over the past fifty years in all sized cities and towns, and with both men and women, young and old.

Below are seven changes in thinking that transformed my life. Every student of the Schuster Center does not experience all seven, but many have.

1.  **From money driven to Purpose Driven**

2.  **From sickness care to Health Care.**

3.  **From dentists' control of treatment choices to patients' freedom to choose.**

4.  **From more is better to less is more.**

**5. From production focus to profitability focus**

**6. From low profit to high profit.**

**7. From five clinical workdays a week to three.**

You are never too young or too old to create a happy, worthwhile life and to create a practice that fulfills your needs and the needs of your patients. What I described is <u>A Better Way to Practice Dentistry</u>. We have chosen to share stories of clients who have learned and applied the model that transformed their lives as ours. You will determine if their lives are better and have been transformed or not.

*"Step up, ye discontented man, pay the price and take it!"*

# Afterward

## *No Man Is an Island*

## A Final Thanks

It is my hope that you read our book from the perspective of learning. Life is a full-time school. If you attend a school and your behavior doesn't change, school is a failure. What I discovered is more important than my story. If you learn, you discover. If you discover and act on truths, your practice and life get better.

There is no such thing as a 'self-made' person. Many people have helped me, guided me, supported me, and loved me. If you pay attention, seek help, and take action, as I did, you make discoveries. Discoveries transform your life from ordinary to extraordinary. It's the Hero's Journey; ordinary people becoming extraordinary because they discovered and acted.

*"Tell me and I forget. Teach me and I remember. Involve me and I learn."*

*- Benjamin Franklin*

I'm thankful for the dentists who sponsored events to engage dentists in creating a better life and practice. Some, such as George Duello, Fred Arnold, Jack King, Ron Roth, Peter Dawson, John

119

Kois, Joan Forrest, and Don Trunkey, referred many dentists to the Schuster Center. Without credible people trusting us, we would not have survived, let alone thrived.

Drs. Fred Arnold, TJ Bolt, Robin Steely, Tim Leary, Mike Robichaux, and Mark Powers spent countless days assisting me in the Schuster Center Continuum and in advanced Programs such as Mastery, Leadership, CEO, and today, Performance Coach. I'm thankful for the Mentors at the Schuster Center, who believed in what we taught, helped me, and guided me. Over the span of forty years, the Schuster Center had three mentor groups and nearly 100 dentists.

Some others to thank:

**Ron Price, CPA.** He called himself a *'financial minister'*. Ron was my personal advisor from 1975 to 2006, when he died. Whenever I faced major issues, we'd meet for several hours for breakfast. He always followed up with notes and suggestions in written form. His advice was priceless. Ron said, *"You show me a person with a financial problem, and I'll show you a person with a spiritual problem."* Ron was an incredible friend and guide to me.

My daughters, **Catherine, Dianne, Christine, and Laura Jo,** all contributed to the Schuster Center. They supported my Vision of the Schuster Center. Laura Jo is still part of the Schuster Center with Dr. Michael Edwards.

**Brenda Penwell,** who trusted me with her career and her life. Brenda was and continues to be a great asset to the Schuster Center. Brenda is a great teacher, a compassionate listener, and a wonderful coach.

**Tony Kong, CPA,** our trusted accountant, followed in Ron's footsteps. **Bruce MacCallum, JD.** who helped us invest our money wisely until he retired. **Jacob Williams,** our current trusted financial advisor.

There are others who believed in and supported the Mission of the Schuster Center.

**James Hollis, Ph.D., Jacob Needleman, Ph.D., Steven Covey, Robert Fritz.**

Especially **Drs. LD Pankey, F. Harold Wirth, and Henry Tanner.** Dr. Pankey trusted me, as one of seven he selected, to carry on his philosophy.

True learning creates a shift in thinking. Learning transforms lives. As you read and re-read the stories in our book, see if you can identify the shifts in thinking that occurred within each dentist's story.

These are some of the shifts Center students have experienced.

- From reacting to creating.

- From me to we.

- From lack of direction to a purpose-driven practice and life.

- From power over patients' treatment choices to helping patients make good choices for themselves.

- From making a small difference to making a big difference in patients' lives.

- From a focus on symptoms of disease to causes of disease.

- From repair focus to prevention focus.

- From high volume to low volume.

- From production to profitability focus.

- From more is more to less is more.

- From doctor-centered to patient-centered.

- From low trust to high trust relationships

- From high stress and anxiety to low stress and anxiety.

- From scarcity attitude to abundance attitude

- From working five days a week to three clinical days a week

- From two weeks off to eight weeks of recreation

- From an ordinary practice to an extraordinary practice and life

Most importantly, I want to thank God for guiding me, assisting me, providing the guides/teachers to allow me to discover and create the Center for Professional Development. Without His help, His guidance, His Interventions, and His creative power, the Vision of the Schuster Center would not have been born, survived, and thrived for fifty years! God willing...it will continue. As Dr. Pankey said to me in 1975, *"Dentists really need what you are planning to do!"*

Lastly, to **Dr. Tim Leary.** When I first started writing the story of how I created the Schuster Model, I went into a deep depression. My friend Dr. Jim Hollis was to write the introduction to the book I was planning. I called Dr. Hollis and apologized to him that I couldn't continue. He responded as only Dr. Hollis could, *"Your soul is telling you not to do this. Stop and do something else."* Writing it alone felt like self-promotion, so I stopped.

When Dr. Leary called me and said he wanted to write a book on how the Schuster Model was created, I said I would if Center clients whose practices and lives had been transformed would also share their stories. This book was Dr. Leary's idea. Tim has completed hundreds of hours of interviewing past Schuster

123

Center students, taping their stories, writing them, getting their edits, re-writing, and having each story approved.

My vision of the Center was to create a place where people could find themselves. I wanted to make a big difference in dentist's lives. The Schuster Center is a *'loaves and fishes story.'* I believe if we could transform the life of one dentist, each dentist could do the same for hundreds, maybe thousands of patients.

We are all indebted to Dr. Tim Leary. What a wonderful human being and outstanding dentist he is. Each of you are also great human beings.

*"You have Infinite Worth and Unlimited Potential for Growth and Development.*

*When given correct information, together with the right support, any worthwhile purpose can be accomplished, provided it is thoroughly planned and properly sequenced."*

I believe the model that I created is correct. Each element of the model is based on principles and proven truths. The Schuster Center provides the right support, for without action, feedback, and support, there is no learning, no discovery, and no transformation. Discovery of a worthwhile purpose is a catalyst for transformation. Anything worthwhile must be thoroughly planned and sequenced properly to achieve the desired outcome. Fifty years of personal application of the Model and forty-plus years of teaching it, witnessing wonderful results of dentists using the model, has proven it works. The model works if you work it.

A strategy is created from a principle. The strategy is applied in a real-life practice environment. Each strategy is a system. Every life and every business is made up of systems. Remember this:

*"Knowledge alone has no power to transform anything.*

*Knowledge organized into useful plans of action (strategies) has power to transform your business or your life."* Adapted from Napoleon Hill's Think and Grow Rich

I leave you with this. I was raised to believe I was born for a reason, a purpose. I believe you were, as well. The day you discover your purpose, your life will be transformed in ways you cannot imagine today.

*Caritas,* Michael

Mike@cfpd.com

563-231-6703

16848 Daisy Trail

Dubuque, Iowa 52001

## Dr. Michael Schuster Timeline

| | |
|---|---|
| 1962 | Graduated from Loras College |
| 1966 | Graduated from Marquette Dental School |
| 1966 | Entered US Navy, completed Navy tour May 1968 |
| 1968 | June, Bought Dr. Walter Barry's equipment & started in practice. |
| 1969 | February, severe bleeding ulcer—hospitalized for seven days. |
| 1969 | Dad introduced me to Maslow and Alfred Adler |

Major discovery—I'd been promoting what people didn't want.

- People wanted NO dentistry.

- Wanted to SPEND as LITTLE money as possible on dentistry.

- Wanted no pain, no abscesses, and as little disease as possible.

- Many had given up on what dentistry had to offer.

| | |
|---|---|
| 1969 | Called Barkley in Macomb—mentored me for two years as I implemented the Disease Control Program |

| 1969 | Made a 'health first' decision for my practice. |
|---|---|
| 1969 | Omer Reed Seminar in Phoenix, Met Bob Zebacknic at a seminar, introduced me to Jim Trask and PEB. |
| 1969 | Tax burden |
| 1969-1975 | Engaged PEB---% budgeting with Money, and Time |
| | A----B----C money, time, staff, patients, procedures |
| | Color coding schedule |
| | Systems Management |
| 1970 | Elliot Simon—Richest Man in Babylon--Principles |
| 1970-1972 | Started Teaching Iowa Dental School |
| 1971-72 | Gnathology Study Club 2 years. Restored 3 cases under supervision. |
| 1971 | Bought property on JFK in Dubuque |
| 1972 | Built building on JFK for group practice. |
| 1972 | LD Pankey Seminar in Ft. Lauderdale. |
| 1972 | Started Pankey Continuum—3rd class. |

| | |
|---|---|
| 1973 | Met Charles Sorenson, helped me hire a team for Dubuque Practice, helped me engage dentists as associates first and partners later. |
| 1973 | Moved practice from Dyersville to Dubuque. |
| 1973 | Finished Pankey Continuum—4 one-week courses. |
| 1973 | Appointed one of 15 Cadres at Pankey. |
| 1974-75 | Taught 24 weeks at Pankey. |
| 1974-1983 | Taught more than 100 weeks at Pankey. |
| 1975 | Met with LD and told him I wanted to start a school where dentists could find themselves. |
| | Defining time in my life. I decided to help others rather than amass more wealth. |
| 1978 | Moved to Scottsdale, AZ. |
| 1978 | Wrote Developing and Managing for Excellence—wrote about the Model I had developed. |
| 1979 | Started new practice in McCormick Ranch—1st dentist in the Ranch. |
| 1979 | Started the Schuster Center-Formalized Schuster Center Practice Development Curriculum. |

| 1980 | First SC workshop at home—Pinnacle Peak. |
|------|------------------------------------------|
| 1981 | First SC class in Michigan. |
| 1979-2010 | Did three seminars a month in the US, Canada, and Puerto Rico. |
| 1983-1989 | Building built on Via Linda for practice and Schuster Center. |
| 1990 | Moved SC to downtown Scottsdale. |
| 1991 | Met Robert Fritz. |
| 1992 | Met Steven Covey. |
| 2001 | Moved to Scottsdale Road. |
| 2003 | New Center Build in 7500 square foot condo in Scottsdale. |

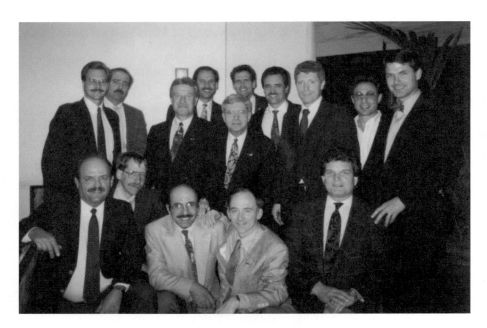

*Dr. Schuster with first Mentor group*
*at the Schuster Center*

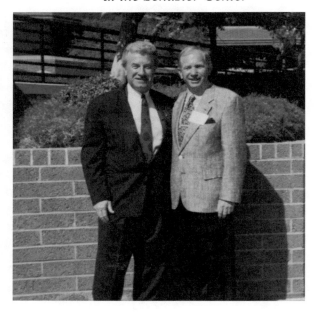

*Dr. Schuster and Dr. Robert Lee*

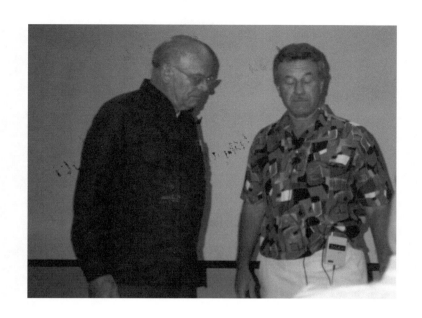

*Dr. Schuster teaching with Dr. Henry Tanner*

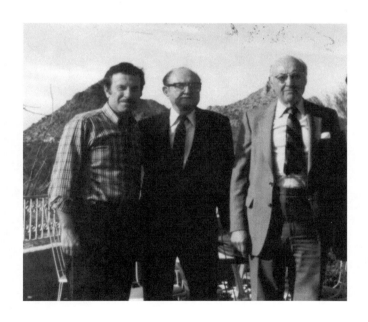

*Dr. Schuster, Dr. LD Pankey, Dr. Harold Wirth*

# Part Three

# Note on the alumni biographies

The Schuster Center (SC) alumni stories were compiled from interviews with each doctor. I told them I wanted to document Dr. Schuster's professional biography and share the good news of the Schuster Model for Practice Success with the profession. Here's how I asked them to prepare.

*Thanks for offering to share your story, and to help chronicle "A Better Way to Practice Dentistry." Your personal experience is unique, but commonalities occur among Schuster alumni that apply to most dentists. We hope readers will find one or more dentist stories that resonate with their own situation and inspire them to engage with the Practice Success Model. The interview will focus on three key areas.*

1. *Why did you decide to engage the SC? What was your life and practice like before you engaged? What frustrations or challenges were you having? What did you hope to gain?*

2. *What happened during SC involvement? How did you feel about what you learned?*

3. *What specific RESULTS were gained from the Schuster Center? I think of two areas. First, tangible, measurable benefits like increased profit or case acceptance, healthier patients, more quadrant dentistry, more time off, etc. Second, what were the*

*subjective, intangible benefits like less stress, more fun, better relationships, peace of mind, etc.*

*I'll record the interview, write an essay, and then have you review it for accuracy and clarity. I look forward to documenting your story in dentistry.*

The interviews were a wonderful experience for me. I became even more passionate about the Schuster Model of Practice Success to generate health and well-being for patients, and fun, prosperity, and purpose for the dental team.

When I considered enrolling in the Management Program at the Schuster Center, the first step was to have a Practice Health Evaluation (PHE) by an analyst. The analyst spent two days in my practice and performed a thorough evaluation. He interviewed me, and all the staff, and assessed the financial, administrative, and clinical aspects of the practice. Then he described the benefits I would gain from the Management program. I was still hesitant about moving forward.

Part of the assessment process was for me to watch a video of a graduate of the program. The video was a pediatric dentist speaking to a class at the Schuster Center. He described how he slowed down his practice, took better care of his patients, improved profitability, and improved his quality of life. It sounded amazing! He emphasized that he was an average guy with no special talents. Rather it was adopting a more professional standard, and the willingness to work ON his practice, not just IN his practice, that led to his success. He stressed that what he learned and the systems he implemented would allow others to achieve similar success if they did the work. The video removed my hesitancy and gave me the confidence to move ahead.

I hope these stories will show dentists who feel trapped, frustrated, or depressed that there is a better way. As Dr. Barkley told Dr. Schuster, "There's nothing wrong with dentistry, but there is something wrong with the way you're doing it."

*Tim Leary*

# Part Three

# Schuster Center Alumni
# Professional Biographies

# Chapter Ten
# Dr. Robin Steely
## Battle Creek, Michigan

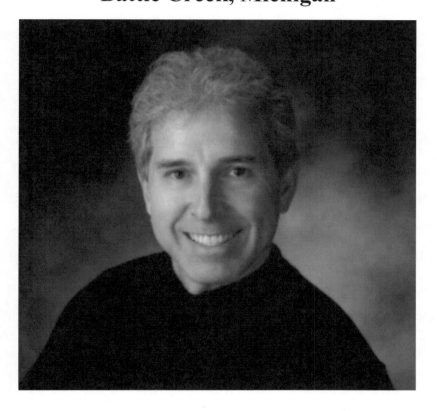

*I'm blessed for all the years I got to work side by side with Dr. Schuster. He is one of the closest mentors I have because of the things I've learned from him, the books he gave me to read, and the investment that he made in me.*

*I'm just here to help people get past disease. If you want to get past disease, then we've got something to talk about.*

## Start-up, Growth and Burnout

I got married right before dental school. I got good with planning so I could have weekends free with my wife. I developed a successful production-based, fee-for-service practice in Battle Creek, Michigan.

I worked with a few practice consultants early in my career. I completed all the courses at the Pankey Institute to develop my clinical skills. I always took lots of continuing education. I just wanted to listen and learn so I could do my best. I think my family upbringing taught me to keep my ego in check and strive for excellence. For example, when I started in practice, I realized I had no knowledge of business concepts, so I took a class from the American Management Society on understanding financial statements.

After ten years into practice, I was frustrated and burned out. I thought I would transition into academic dentistry, so I condensed my work schedule down to three and a half days and enrolled in a master's program in Oral-Facial Pain. One day a week for thirty-five weeks, I traveled to Lexington, KY for the course. A long-time friend from school, Sharon Dickerson, encouraged me to enroll in the Schuster Center Management Program. She thought it would help me get control of my practice and achieve greater professional satisfaction. We had closely followed each other's careers from dental school. I bought the practice of my family dentist, and she took over her father's dental practice. We both completed Pankey courses.

I had a long talk with Dr. Schuster after one of his seminars. Based on that conversation, I went home and dropped my consultant. It turns out more production wasn't my problem. What I really wanted was less stress, more satisfaction, better relationships with my patients, and more time to connect with people.

An analyst from the Schuster Center performed a Practice Health Evaluation, which is a comprehensive assessment of the driving forces in a dental practice—finance, marketing, sales, staff, organization, facility, mix of services, etc. After that, I signed on for the one-year Management program. My staff was supportive and understood that I wanted to make some changes.

The Schuster Center helped me recapture *why* I went to dental school. I'd wanted to be a dentist since the eighth grade. I have good hands and good eyes, and I enjoy the technical stuff. I have fun with lab work and the creative aspect of dentistry, such as figuring out how to solve dental problems. In dental school, I looked for patients with severe problems who needed extensive repair. I finished my requirements early with a base of only fifteen patients because they all needed extensive treatment.

## A Better Way to Practice - Transformation

Implementing the Schuster Model allowed me to get my life under control. We reworked all aspects of the practice, and we wrote policies and systems to focus on improving relationships, seeing one patient at a time, and promoting health rather than repairing disease. The transition was a lot of work, but that's on purpose. We figured out a schedule and worked through all the systems. Following are the major highlights over time:

I completed the one-year Management Program in 2003. But the benefits were big, and I stayed connected to the Schuster Center. I've made four trips a year to Arizona, many with my team, for sixteen years.

I was able to improve and really apply my clinical skills and advanced training.

I'm more relaxed, open, and relationship-driven after Schuster training. I have time for building relationships with patients and the team. My team is long-term: I've employed one person for 33 years, another for 16 years, and two hygienists for 25 years.

I decreased stress in the practice, and increased profitability. Last year we worked ten days less but maintained the same level of profit. My team tracks the numbers, and office overhead is stable between 52-54%.

I'm more relaxed about practice numbers now. I prefer to track how many complete cases I finish per year, instead of worrying about daily and monthly production.

We've gone from eight staff members to five, and from three assistants to one.

I've gone from seeing twelve patients a day to 6-7 a day.

I've improved my leadership skills. It helped me develop my team and let them run the show. Better communication helps me coach patients to health and explain the benefits of long-term solutions to their problems.

New patients are waiting six months to get into the practice. I can't see more than four to five new patients/month because more than that and I can't keep up with the dentistry. The bottom line is that I see fewer patients, but each patient chooses more complete care.

I work 3.5 days per week. I have full staff Monday to Wednesday. On Thursdays, I work only in the morning with one hygienist. The time is reserved for new patients, Review of Findings consults, surgery, administrative tasks, and working ON my practice, not in the practice.

The Dental Fitness Program is key to our success. It helps patients actively control decay and gum disease, and it helps them make better long-term choices regarding treatment.

My new patient process has an open agenda. I don't put heavy sales pressure on people to accept treatment.

I help patients figure out what led to their oral breakdown. I use a simple brochure to help them understand the progress of the disease. I have them co-diagnose where they are on the pyramid of health regarding their teeth, gums, and bite. Then, at the Review of Findings consultation we build a new recipe for health that will get them the outcome they want. I've gotten away from being the expert and telling people what to do. Instead, we have a collaborative agreement on the target, what they want for their health and their smile long term, and the strategy to help them get there.

I use a template for the patient's Review of Findings report. It's fast and easy to edit for each patient, and the staff collates the printed copy with the patient's photos. It's an overall view of their oral health, not a detailed description of treatment and fees.

It's rewarding to work with people and not push them to want what I want. I tell them, "I'm just here to help you get past disease. If you want to get past disease, then we have something to talk about."

After some years, I became a mentor at the Schuster Center. I helped Dr. Schuster multiple times to teach the three-day New Patient Experience class. Mentoring reinforces my values and beliefs in relationship care. It keeps them fresh and relevant.

I continued practice refinement and personal growth with Dr. Schuster via the Performance Coach Program. Eight of the original ten doctors are still in the group. We have been meeting three times/year for fifteen years. We have two group phone calls every month. Now I help mentor other dentists in Performance Coach (PC). It's been really good, and it's allowed me to share and teach. Teaching helps me know my stuff. Younger dentists see what we mentors have done, and it helps them know if I did it, then they can do it too. My PC colleagues are my best friends in dentistry.

I've been blessed to meet people who share my values. They mentored me, coached me, and took me into different areas of whole-body health. I took courses from Brad Bale (Beat the Heart Attack Gene), and Tom Nabors at OralDNA, and I have a better understanding of total physical, mental, and emotional health.

## Final Thoughts

I feel like I moved into the second half of life mindset early in my career, instead of waiting until my sixties. I let go of the production model for practice success and treatment acceptance. I try to focus on taking care of people and helping them prevent disease. I've saved enough money to retire and maintain my standard of living.

My faith is important, and my wife played a huge part in my success. She's very open and relationship-driven, and she cares about people. She has the gift of hospitality and that's how she always cared for her hygiene patients. I was the driven one. If I get upset, she'll just listen. Ten minutes later I've blown past it, and then we can talk about it.

I'm in a local study club. The newer dentists tend to ignore the importance of leadership skills, effective communication, and relationship building. They all think they need dental insurance or else patients will leave their practice. It's transaction dentistry.

Mike Robichaux in Louisiana is a friend and Schuster mentor. He says, "Some people have the chip." In PC we look for younger dentists who have the chip. If they've got it, there is no way they're getting away from us. We grab them and say, "You're going to do this." Some are like sponges wanting to help patients and practice this way. Helping these dentists is really fun! It forces me to learn it, know it, and practice it.

*Dr. Robin Steely has a fee-for-service practice in Battle Creek, Michigan. He graduated from Michigan Dental School. He and a partner purchased the practice of his family dentist in 1982. He bought out his partner two years later. His practice is mostly adults and some families. His wife is a retired hygienist, and he has three grown children who have all gone into the healthcare profession.*

# Chapter Eleven
# Dr. John Korolewski
## Sheboygan, Wisconsin

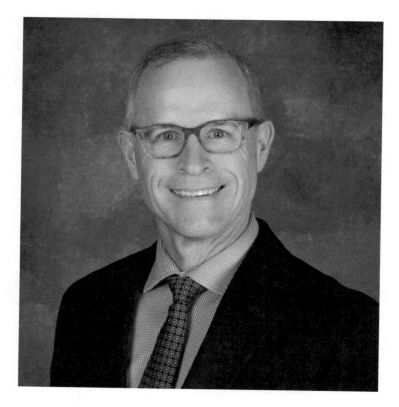

*I realized I didn't even know what I didn't know. I was really uncomfortable.*

*I came to the Schuster Center to get control of money and improve case acceptance, but I got much more. We get a lot of technical training, and we think—you know I'm a doctor and I'm smart. It hampered me and I lost humility. Here's my favorite joke. Do you know the difference between God and a doctor? Even God doesn't think he's a doctor.*

## Startup – Growth, Stress, and Frustration

For several years I built a high-stress, high-production office in Sheboygan, WI, patterned after the corporate dentistry model I learned at Midwest Dental. I equated busyness with success, and more new patients and more patient visits meant more revenue. But I was feeling burned out and beat up treating a high volume of patients every day and rendering piecemeal, repair dentistry. One day I came home and said to my wife, "I'm going to have a heart attack."

Later I would learn, working with Mike Schuster, that I got exactly what I created. I thought a high-production, high-amped practice was the way to go. But I really wanted to slow down, do more quadrant dentistry, and increase my hourly production. At age forty-three I was a half million dollars in debt with my house and practice. I had no sense of accumulating wealth. I didn't understand the difference between high revenue and being wealthy. I wasn't confident about achieving financial independence.

I was attracted to the Schuster Center by the tagline on their website, "The Business School for Dentists." I purchased the book on Preventive Dentistry by Bob Barkley, and a DVD series by Dr. Schuster called "Truth in Selling." I learned I didn't know what I didn't know. I was really uncomfortable. I thought, I don't know much about this Schuster guy, but I can't stop listening to these DVDs. Previously, I believed the only way I was going to do big treatment plans was if I sold them, closed them, and so on. But it wasn't working.

I completed the curriculum at Pankey Institute and was exposed to doing more complete care. I learned more about occlusion, diagnosing, and treating patients with an unstable bite. I began to recognize early signs of bite problems. But I had this cognitive dissonance. I didn't feel Pankey taught me enough strategies about how to move people forward.

I was able to help patients who were in survival, ie. their mouths were really broken down and they knew they were in trouble. But I was failing with all the other people. I saw patients with early signs of disease, but they didn't have significant disability yet. I couldn't move them forward. I had a basement full of study models on them and I usually heard, "I'll think about it." I was really left wanting. I realized I didn't have all the pieces yet of the practice I wanted.

In 2010 I had a Practice Health Evaluation by Korbin Reeves from the Schuster Center. He reviewed the numbers for my practice and discussed where and how I could improve. I wanted to get firm control of money, determine if I was on track for financial independence, and achieve better case acceptance for complete dentistry.

I remember sitting at the table with my wife across from Korbin. He spun around his laptop and showed us the tuition fee for the one-year Management Program at the Schuster Center. I was thinking I need to think about this. But then my wife spoke up before I could. She said, "Well OK, we're doing it!" I was worried about the cost. She was worried about my health and figured the price was worth it.

## A Different Model of Practice - Transformation

I started the Management Program in 2011, with training, monthly reports, and phone calls from a Support Coach at the SC. I had two-hour team meetings every two weeks, and progressively we restructured practice for less stress, more quadrant dentistry, more profit, and better health for patients. I implemented written policies/systems to run all aspects of the practice—percentage budgeting, block scheduling, hygiene visits, fee setting, the new patient process (NPP), collections, monitoring stats, etc.

I decided that the only way to evaluate if this model was effective, was I had to embrace all of it. I met people who would only do parts of the model, and maybe they were successful with that, but I was determined to add all of it. I wanted to capture all that Schuster's model had to offer.

Initially, I was pulling staff along. Later they told me how grateful they were that we were so organized. They recognized the benefits, and we gained confidence. Being organized we had more time to devote to patients. There was less time wasted on not knowing how to do something, or figuring out whose job it was. My team enjoyed sharing our progress with specialists and other general dentists.

I developed a budget and a spreadsheet for tracking key performance indicators called a Profitability Management Controller Report (PMCR.) We reviewed the PMCR monthly at a team meeting. It was more useful than expense reports from my accountant.

After a while, I knew exactly how many days I could take off during the year, what kind of fee increase I could do, and how much hygiene demand I really had. All the decisions that I needed to make were based on accurate numbers. I knew exactly what the real profit was, my overhead, and how to assess debt. Over a decade I achieved the following results.

For the ten years, 2010-20, my net worth increased 8-9 times. Saving money felt good, and it became a positive reinforcement. I was paying down debt and building wealth, net worth, and my solvency account. It gave me confidence and peace of mind to know I was on track.

I started to have a better relationship with money. I set the goal to have financial independence for retirement by age 62. Then I just put the plan in place and didn't worry about it. In fact, I retired earlier than I anticipated due to a neck injury. But financially we were able to do it. No hardship or struggle.

We went from 4 days to 3.5 days per week. Staff size stayed the same: 6 days of hygiene, 1 full-time and 1 part-time, 2 FT assistants, and 1 front desk coordinator.

Revenues stayed the same but net profit went up. I worked less and had more profit.

I took Mike's advice on buying toys. Any toys that we bought we paid for with cash.

Increased profit allowed me to fund retirement. I went from sole proprietor to LLC. I was able to decrease taxes and set money aside. The money was there previously, but my tax structure wasn't as beneficial as it could have been.

I developed a hybrid practice of repair dentistry and complete dentistry. Most mornings were quadrant dentistry, and afternoons were consults, a mix of operative, and shorter visits.

The New Patient process became the focal point of the practice. It became the thing that singled me out most in my community. I enjoyed espousing my values, being an attentive listener, and developing better communication skills. I remember Mike saying,

*"Say what you believe and the more you'll believe it. The more you believe it, the more your patients will believe it, and the more your staff will believe it."*

That became my mantra interacting with patients, letting them know what I believed about patient care, about health, and about them having control over their health. I was no longer rambling and pushing people. It was being together with each person in the new patient process—trying to discover something that they may not be aware of, what they wanted, why they wanted it, what they valued and why, what they saw for the future, what their concerns were, and what they were afraid of. Also, what prevented them from going forward, getting them to think of things they hadn't thought of, or weren't able to share with previous dentists?

The puzzle of discovery almost became more rewarding than the clinical puzzle and figuring out how to fix them! That's the part I'm going to miss most about dentistry, sitting down with the patient.

Patients got actively involved (rather than passively having their teeth cleaned or decay repaired.) The Dental Fitness Program became integral to our practice. The patient has responsibility, we have a responsibility, and the body has a responsibility. Health is not something that is bought, or given away, it's something that you must actively work at. People who got healthy periodontally, were better listeners when it came to discussing restorative options, tooth wear, and jaw joint health. But it didn't work well the other way around at all.

## Final Thoughts

My biggest obstacle to accepting this was an incorrect belief. I thought all patients wanted corporate-type care. I wondered if patients would be attracted to this type of office. What about Google, Instagram, big signs, and marketing? I worried that the Schuster Model is all fine and good, but I need more new patients because the guy on Delta Dental is seeing 25 new patients. I took it on a leap of faith that there were people out there looking for this and it turned out to be true. I put my philosophy out there, what my values were, so people could see it on the website or hear it from another patient. I'm still impressed when patients come in and say "I didn't know there were dentists doing anything like this. I'm not treated like a number."

If you build a relationship-based, patient-centered, slowed-down practice there are people attracted to it and who are seeking that. I think they give up after a while and they just stop looking.

Even in the small city of Sheboygan, Wisconsin, I had enough people that I would not have run out of new patients and dentistry to do. Whereas before I was. I was a repair dentist trying to attract people like I was different. People would come in and see that I was running fast and that I was nice, but I wasn't in their network. The guy across the street is also nice, and he runs fast, and he's in their network. So, they weren't seeing a difference. But when I adopted a health-centered, patient-centered model— the way we answered the phone to the New Patient Process, how we did that, and how we presented treatment—we no longer looked like anybody else!

I regarded tuition for the Schuster Center as a cost of doing business. It's like clinical training after dental school, but training for financial, organizational, leadership, communication, and business skills.

## Unexpected Benefits

The new patient process was so much fun it became a hobby.

I completed more restorative training at the Stewart Center in Texas and learned how to do conservative, non-invasive complete dentistry with matrix-guided, composite addition. I completed forty-five full mouth rejuvenations over five years and served as faculty at the Stewart Center. The improved clinical skills were great, but it was my patient-centered, new patient process, and focus on health, skills I learned from the Schuster Center, that helped patients accept complete dentistry. Teaching the Schuster Model to other dentists is something I never anticipated, but I found it fun and rewarding.

Another unexpected benefit of the Schuster Center was this notion of the two worlds we live in. It's led me on a journey beyond dentistry. My wife and I together have explored many different things outside the practice for meaning, fulfillment, and growth. I wouldn't be at this point if it wasn't for working with Mike Schuster. I wasn't going to the Schuster Center to discover what spiritual opportunities might be out there to develop, but that was one of the results of it.

*Dr. John Korolewski retired in 2022. He had a fee-for-service practice in Sheboygan, WI, a small town of 50,000 north of Milwaukee. The community is mostly blue-collar and farming. He graduated from Marquette Dental School in 1986 and completed a hospital general practice residency in Madison. He worked as an associate in Milwaukee for four years, and then a few years in*

*Manitowoc for Midwest Dental, a corporate dental group. He purchased his practice in Sheboygan in 1999, where he worked until retirement.*

# Chapter Twelve
# Dr. Sue Vetter
### Seattle, Washington

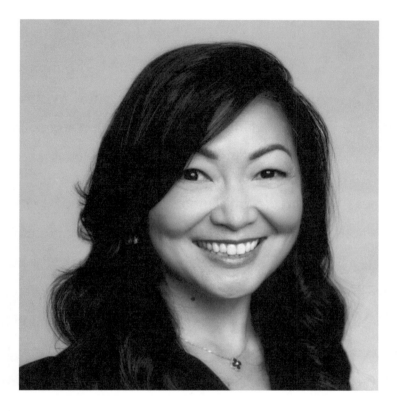

*Hands down the Schuster Center and OBI are the best programs I did. The Schuster Center for my leadership, business, and spiritual development, and OBI for my clinical skills. But I always tell dentists to do the Schuster Center first so you can leverage your clinical skills.*

*I like one-to-one, small group, hands-on learning like that offered at the Schuster Center and OBI. That type of learning makes you accountable for the knowledge and delivering all the skills you learned.*

## Aloha Beginnings

My parents were first-generation immigrants from Korea. I grew up on Oahu amidst family drama that made life challenging and uncertain. It was crazy! My husband says I should go on Oprah. I was told to study hard, be a good student, and obey my parents. They told me when I turned eighteen, I would be on my own. So, I realized at a young age I would be responsible for my future. I left home at fifteen and moved in with my grandmother so I could attend a high school in Honolulu that had a high acceptance rate to college.

I was first attracted to dentistry in high school. I cold called several dental offices within walking distance of my grandmother's apartment. I offered to volunteer so I could confirm my interest. I got a part-time job in an office sterilizing instruments. Eventually, I worked as a chairside assistant and front office receptionist. I experienced the dynamics of a group dental practice, and I really enjoyed the doctor-patient interactions. Patient relationships were more personal than when I worked in a hospital. I'm introverted, but I like working with people and creating a positive experience for them under the umbrella of professional service.

## Mainland Education, Start-Up, and Break Point

I went to college and dental school at the University of Washington. My parents didn't help pay for undergraduate or dental school. I paid tuition and expenses by working part-time as a waitress and a bartender. I borrowed some money from a mentor, a previous employer, to buy dental supplies. After graduation, I worked for a year as an associate in a large insurance-driven practice. That experience caused me a lot of anxiety and stress. I learned what I didn't like, i.e., making patients wait, not having the right equipment, and working long hours without a break. Further, I was always shifting between four operatories—two doctor rooms and checking two rooms of hygiene patients.

In 2000, At the age of 27, I purchased a practice in a Seattle suburb for $740,000. 100% of the practice price was financed and my monthly loan payment was $11,000. The interest rate then was 9.5%! After seven years a crisis ensued. Stress was getting unbearable. I had two mortgages. My husband's job was unstable, and his income was inconsistent. I hated being in debt, and I was bleeding income from the practice to pay expenses for our home, our children, and my in-laws.

I was getting burned out and thinking, is this all there is? I don't like it! Something is missing! I didn't have enough tools in my toolbox. I needed better clinical skills and leadership skills to develop my team. I was almost paralyzed with worry. Would I have to work until I was a hundred years old? I realized I needed to make a change and focus on my practice. My husband understood and he was supportive. I didn't need huge wealth, but I had to get control of my finances for stability and security.

I was a member of the Seattle Study Club. In 2007 I decided to attend the annual symposium in California. The focus was entirely on the business side of dentistry. Top practice management experts from around the country were lecturing. I was feeling emotional and vulnerable at that time. On top of family turbulence in my life and financial stress, I'd just learned my grandmother had a stroke and was going to hospice. I listened to the experts and took plenty of notes, but the lectures seemed scattershot and incomplete. Then Mike Schuster began his presentation, and I had an epiphany.

It was like a scene in a movie. All the lights went dim, and it was just me and Dr. Schuster. Is he talking to me? Does he know my troubles? Does he know my concerns? Oh my god, I can't believe this! Everything he said was like, oh my god that's me! I used to listen to classical music, and it was like hearing a beautiful aria. I thought I needed to learn more about this.

Compared to the other advisors, Mike Schuster probed the soul of the doctor. In addition, the soul of the practice needed to be studied, i.e., what's going on inside and is not visible. It's not just about what's on the surface, like production, collection, and new patients. Of course, those are important. But they aren't separate from purpose, meaning, professional service, and career satisfaction. It's all connected and interrelated!

## Schuster Center Magic and Benefits

Dr. Schuster helped me take my focus off worry and direct that focus onto developing myself, my team, my patients, and my practice. I'd studied some with Spear, Dawson, and Kois, and I was on a track to learn more about occlusion. I knew some things and I had some great ideas, but my practice was fragmented. I needed help with structure and organization. I'd purchased a good practice, but I wanted to design the practice and office culture to fit my values, preferences, and personality.

I got control over money, and time. In addition, I got the practice organized properly according to the style of practice I wanted, not the style I inherited from the previous owner. Template scheduling was a big help, especially in a small practice to promote an even flow of the day. I learned a subtle but big, important point. It's more effective to have the office team centered on something external. For example, it's not just that "Dr. wants this." No, it's "the practice wants this." The Schuster Center helps dentists separate the practice from the doctor, and have it be a separate entity so that the team understands that.

It's like successful marriages. If you tend to the marriage as a separate entity, not focusing on the individuals, it works out better. It keeps me in check if I get frustrated. It helps me be more objective and less emotional with decision-making. I can be less fearful and take more risks when I need to.

We have periodic staff meetings and annual team retreats. I learned how to delegate. I'm stable and friendly at work. I'm not moody, but I have high expectations of people. I learned to distinguish between my role as a business owner and my role as a clinician in the practice. I liked learning to understand practice metrics or key performance indicators. Understanding the numbers allows me to know immediately what's really happening in the practice and determine the source of the problems. I can look at the numbers objectively, and it removes most of the emotion from tough decisions.

A valuable team member said to me one day "You know Sue you have to move and think like everyone is replaceable." It's true. I trained many people, and they always message me saying "Thank you so much and I remember all that you taught me." I invested in those people out of pure care and love for them. I was thinking at the time that they would give back to me and the practice in equal measure. In a way they did, but not 100%, and not in the way that most doctors expect it to occur. That was frustrating. It takes time and maturity to understand why. They have no liability, no financial investment, and no equity in your practice.

Creating policies and systems of organization was hard work but very effective. I'm happy I made time for that. But we don't do much of that now. We're beyond putting out fires every day, and haphazard problem-solving.

Expanding and developing the new patient process has been extraordinary for the practice, financially, emotionally, and professionally. I like getting to know patients and creating a high touch learning experience for them. I get the new patient from the front, and we have a conversation first. I focus on building rapport, getting their history, and understanding their expectations. It's not scripted. I allow for a free flow of conversation. In case they've had bad experiences previously I avoid giving them bad news early on.

Then we go into the operatory and I do the exam in a co-discovery manner. Seattle is a demographic where good communication is key. The exam has three parts—gums, teeth, and chewing system. I collect all data and records. Then, unless I see something that needs urgent attention I tell the patient, "I'll review everything on my own time." They come back for a consultation which I piggyback with a hygiene appointment. I'll let them know their periodontal and caries status. Based on their experience and how they present that day we see where they want to go and how we can work together. If we need more time to discuss their chewing system, then I'll bring them back for a second consultation/review of the findings.

## Practice Maturity—Peace, Balance, and Profitability

After the Schuster Center Management program, I stayed connected to the Schuster Center for twenty years with Performance Coach. The long-term friendships with other like-minded dentists have been tremendous for me. It's helped me stay on track with my vision, keep reading good books, and continue to develop myself and the practice.

I see patients three days a week and spend one day a week on administrative tasks and lab work. It's been that way for twenty-two years. I work from 7 am to 3:30 pm and take a half hour for lunch. I don't bring work home from the office, and I'm not afraid to take time off. I average twelve workdays/month, and I take a week off every three months. I see one column of patients when I work, and the practice has five days of hygiene/week. I do big restorative cases on Mondays when there is no hygiene. Of course, I change the work schedule as needed to make room for fun stuff. I like the balance between my work life and my personal life. I don't want to have multiple practices and all the stress that goes with it. I prefer spending quality time with my family and friends rather than pushing for more production.

Profitability is better. I learned to pay myself first and save money. I'll save money first and then I'll buy things I can afford. After learning about the five engines of growth, I can look at the practice numbers and know where to focus my energy—time, money, organization, people, or technology. The Schuster Center helped me remove fear, and stress around money, time, and organization, and be kinder to myself as a clinician. I don't have many stressful patients now.

I dropped Delta in 2011. It was pivotal for me and for the practice. Without what I learned at the Schuster Center I wouldn't have had the confidence to become insurance independent. I'd been with the Schuster Center for three years at that time. Also, it was the last year of my loan payment. The Schuster Center helped me hunker down, pay off my debts, and position myself to be in a good place to withstand any loss of patients.

I remember thinking about the worst-case scenario. I read Gus Lee's book, *Courage: The Backbone of Leadership*. I visualized losing all my patients and going bankrupt. I told myself it would be embarrassing and disappointing, but I could live with it. I still have skills, I can get a job, be an associate, and I can still earn. If I'm going to sink this ship at least I'll be the captain. I'm going to do it fighting so there are no regrets and no doubts.

Currently, many dentists are trying to get out of network with PPOs and I get invited to speak on the topic by study clubs, the dental school, and dental societies. I like to help doctors think differently about their practice. There is an alternative to a high-stress, insurance-driven practice. Many dentists feel like they don't have an option and that's a dreadful story. They get stuck in a treadmill practice they don't like because of high lifestyle expenses.

## OBI Faculty, Teaching, and Giving Back to Dentistry

Dr. Schuster introduced me to the Foundation for Bioesthetic Dentistry (OBI) for advanced training in occlusion and restorative dentistry. OBI reinforced what I learned at the Schuster Center. It's inspiring to be around other high-achieving, dedicated dentists. Those dentists impressed me with their calmness and humility, and their friendships have been huge. Their approach to patients is about caring, health, and wellness.

Dr. Benson, the former president of OBI saw something in me that I didn't even see in myself. I'm my own toughest critic. I can take on too much responsibility and try to do too much. Dr. Benson said to me "You are a star, and you shine so bright, but you don't seem to see it. You don't seem to look up and see that about

166

yourself. We need more women in OBI. I hope that you will help and want to teach."

I like one-to-one, small group, hands-on learning like that offered at the Schuster Center and OBI. That type of learning makes you accountable for the knowledge and delivering all the skills you learned. If you don't workshop the curriculum and do what's taught in a supportive environment, then you're not going to continue in your practice after getting a certificate. I didn't see that type of teaching in other clinical and management programs.

Of all the advanced clinical courses I've taken—Dawson, Spear, Kois, and OBI—OBI has given the most return on my investment. I always tell other doctors, to do the Schuster Center first so that they can leverage the investment they've made in their clinical training. That's how you get advanced restorative care "off the shelf" and get the best bang for your CE dollars.

I teach a course at OBI with Dr. Mike Edwards. Teaching has helped me grow my leadership skills and reinforce my clinical skills. Public speaking is not my thing. I can be a director, but not an actor. It's still a hurdle for me but I'm figuring it out. I try to do something uncomfortable every day to develop my confidence. Of course, my journey has had hiccups and hurdles, but I would do it all over again.

*Dr. Vetter has a patient-centered, fee-for-service practice in Seattle, WA. She obtained her BS and DDS degrees from the University of Washington where she remains an affiliate associate professor. She is an alumna of the Dawson Academy, Kois Center, Schuster Center for Professional Development, OBI Foundation for Bioesthetic Dentistry, and The Mastery Company. Dr. Vetter is a faculty member of the OBI and serves on its board.*

*Originally from Honolulu, Hawaii, Dr. Vetter has made Seattle her home since 1991. Dr. Vetter, her husband, and their two children enjoy spending time together cooking, dancing, or playing outdoors.* *https://www.suevetter.com*

# Chapter Thirteen
# Dr. Mike Edwards, CEO of the Schuster Center
## Union, Missouri

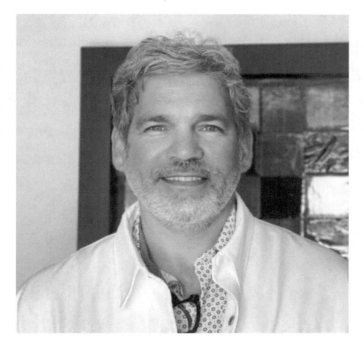

*It was a moment of truth in the car that day. I realized there was no way
I wanted to work like that for the next forty years. There had to be a
better way. Thankfully, there is! That's what I want to share...*

*It's difficult to practice dentistry at a mastery level without a mastery
team to back you up.*

*Dentists keep taking clinical courses thinking. "Dentistry is what
I do know so if I can learn more, then I can produce more."*

*But it's not true.*

## Breakdown and a Moment of Truth

I was an equal partner in a busy two-doctor office. I was sitting in my car before walking into the office one morning. I didn't want to get out of my car. I'd had the practice for a year and already, I was worn out. Every day I had an hour commute to and from the office. Because we offered evening hours for patient convenience, some days I didn't get home until 9:30 pm. Then I had to be at the office by 7:15 the next morning, ready to go with a busy schedule. I worked five days/week and every other Saturday. It was exhausting. How had I ended up like this? It's not the picture I envisioned while attending dental school.

It was a moment of truth in the car that day. I realized there was no way I wanted to do that for the next forty years. There had to be a better way. Thankfully, there is! That's what I want to share.

## Startup

I grew up surrounded by dentists. My best friend's dad was a dentist, and our next-door neighbor was a dentist. In college I considered studying to be a veterinarian, then a physician, but settled on dental medicine. I was attracted to dentistry because I didn't have to do a residency, and I could still practice a type of medicine and treat people and I wasn't going to be thirty-five when I was finished with schooling. At that time, I didn't realize a health professional never really stops learning.

Further, I wanted to be my own boss. I grew up in a steel town and worked in steel factories during summer vacations. It was brutal. I worked by the blazing hot coke ovens in extreme heat protective gear. It was intense and dangerous. It was good money for a young man, but my co-workers considered it a death sentence. Along with dangerous work conditions, I didn't like the adversarial relationship between the unions and management. It was counterproductive and would routinely cause the mill to file bankruptcy only to reopen a few months or years later, which would shortly afterward result in the union going on strike. It was a vicious cycle.

After graduation from dental school, I worked as an associate dentist for nine months. The owner dentist was former faculty at Washington University in St Louis, where he taught occlusion. He wasn't in the office much, and I soon realized I wanted to build my own practice where I could do more restorative dentistry. I don't like being under the control of someone else, so I wanted my own dental practice.

I found a large two-doctor practice to buy and enlisted a dental school classmate to be my partner in the purchase. The

171

practice had thirteen staff members, and the owner's doctors had been through the Schuster Center Management program. They had implemented some systems of the Schuster Model, but I didn't understand why or how they organized operations to control finances, time, and patient management. I somewhat looked at production and collection, and I was paid a salary — that is what I knew.

The practice was high volume, and we were busy. We had 5-10 emergencies every day, and most care was same-day treatment. As mentioned, I was working five days and one evening a week, and every other Saturday. In addition, I had an hour commute each way to the office from home. After a year I was burned out and couldn't continue. So, we signed up for the Schuster Center's Practice Management program. It was a leap of faith. I didn't know what to expect, but I knew I was unhappy with what we had, and I had to decrease stress. The tuition was $40,000, which seemed crazy because nothing in dentistry cost that much at the time, not even digital radiography equipment.

## Schuster Center Management and Mastery Programs

The analyst from the Schuster Center performed a Practice Health Evaluation (PHE.) He told us we needed to get finances under control and our overhead was too high. Also, we needed to address interpersonal conflict between my partner and me. The office environment was dysfunctional. Staff had splintered into two camps, each loyal to one doctor. Problems were usually blamed on one side or the other.

During the management year, we got finances under control. There was a big increase in profit because we lowered overhead from 75-80% to about 55%. The staff decreased from thirteen to eight, and we saved enough money to pay off the total tuition. I was especially intrigued by the new patient process. I concentrated on relationship building, trust, and independent health to help patients address the causes of disease. We already had a structure in place for a two-visit new patient exam/consult, but I didn't understand how to make it effective.

I was encouraged by progress in the first year and I immediately signed up for the two-year Mastery program, which has since been replaced by a similar program, Performance Coach (PC.) Mastery was designed to help the doctor move the practice closer to his or her ideal vision, improve the health and well-being of the doctor and the office team, and improve the health of patients in the practice. I took the Mastery philosophy to heart with nutrition, exercise, stress control, and careful analysis of my blood chemistry. I got into the best shape of my life and was even doing triathlons.

During the second year of Mastery, I really started to love dentistry, and that love grew even more over the next decade. The improved level of care for our patients was in alignment with my core values.

We implemented the Dental Fitness Program to empower people to gain control over bacterial gingivitis, periodontitis, and decay, and create health. The idea is to help patients help themselves and avoid tooth loss or invasive surgery for periodontal disease. Later on, I got involved with Mark Powers who developed the computerized version of the Dental Fitness Program, and I did some teaching to help dentists with their new patient process.

My partner and I started advanced clinical training, and we quickly completed the Dawson Academy and the Piper program. We were go-getters in the course. We read the manuals, watched all the videos, and practiced with each other and the team so we could quickly get competent. Then we would show up to class and fill in the gaps in our learning or lack of experience. I'm surprised when I see doctors enroll in training or management programs and they don't do the homework to get the biggest bang for their buck.

## Benefits

The Management and Mastery programs enabled me to get control of money, decrease overhead, and increase profit. I paid off my dental school and practice debt. I was able to send my three children to private school, which cost $250,000 each. I started funding a retirement plan and a savings account for the practice. After seven years I bought out my partner. Over the years we moved apart as I embraced a health-centered philosophy of care and she stayed with the more common insurance-based, repair style of care.

With Dental Fitness we measured the health of our patients. I always focused on helping patients avoid full mouth rehabilitation. My training early on was to learn to do comprehensive restorative dentistry, but also find ways to help people avoid complex repairs.

I have a long-term, loyal staff. Not all dentists understand the power of a dynamic team. I experienced it early on, and I strived to maintain it during my career. I like to create stewards on the team so that everyone understands the direction of the practice. Then we can move from stewardship to accountability. They understand why tracking stats is important. They understand the big picture and support me to enhance profitability. They understand how each person's role supports the whole. That's a big thing for me. It's always about the people.

Dr. Schuster told us early in the Management program that 80% of our success would come from the relationships we have, from our ability to form relationships, and from our ability to lead.

The other 20% of success is from organized systems and our technical ability. For ten years I spent most of my study time developing that part of my psyche, my ability to form relationships, to quickly identify a person's values, to build rapport, to find out the outcome people want, and the Drivers of that outcome. Then I switched and focused heavily on the technical side of dentistry.

Over the years the size of my practice has varied. At one time I had two practice locations and two associates, a periodontist and a pedodontist. I operated that way for ten years. I spent two days a week at each office, and the practice manager traveled with me. Now I have one practice location with a pediatric dentist here one day a week. It's a family practice with 600 active patients. I never done any advertising other than a website and posting a few things on Facebook. Recently, about 20% of my new patients are from out of state. Amazing.

I have an associate pediatric dentist who has been with me for the last fifteen years. He is here a few days a month. He was a Marine (I think you are always a Marine), and we enjoyed discussing the team and office functioning and efficiencies. He taught me this phrase: our team "takes appropriate action in the absence of orders." The goal is for your people to understand what you want, and why you want it. Then they think the same way you do, and they will take action on your behalf, without you there.

An unexpected, wonderful benefit of the Schuster Center has been the people I've met and studied with during my career. I met a new network of people moving in a similar direction. It's hard to overstate the importance of spending time with like-minded people who value personal growth. Except for a few months, I've been connected with Mike Schuster and Schuster Center mentors and alumni since the Management year.

Here's an example of what happened when I got serious about my vision At Dr. Schuster's recommendation. Some of the early books we read at the Center and some lectures at annual meetings allowed me to get to know Robert Fritz. In time, I enrolled in the Robert Fritz's Structural Certification Coaching Program. It was intense training and study over a five-year period. We worked side by side with world-class musicians, filmmakers, and creative artists—it's the deep end of the pool of the creative process. It had nothing to do with dentistry, but everything to do with structure. I learned to use structural tension to create the outcome I want in many aspects of business and life. It's a stepwise process. First, know clearly what I want to create, how life will be different after I create it, what the elements of that, and what the drivers are. Then I establish the reality of where I am now. I must be able to write down the outcome I want and visualize so strongly that the universe conspires to help me bring it about.

After Mastery I joined a Performance Coach group that I'm still involved with. In 2013 we hired Mike Schuster for a two-day course focused on the new patient experience. It was a turning point for me. Prior to the retreat, I was struggling with patient acceptance for complete treatment. That weekend I learned the importance of making time for a sequence of appointments and letters to build value for optimal restorative care. It's so much easier to get overhead down to 40-50% when you are doing comprehensive dentistry.

Dr. Schuster then referred me to OBI. It's a multi-course comprehensive residency program in occlusion and restorative dentistry. The OBI biology-centered methodology is a great fit with the Schuster Model focuses on controlling the causes of dental disease and oral-facial breakdown. I went through all the OBI courses in consecutive sequences over four years. Because of my SC training, I had multiple patients ready and eager to go when I proposed comprehensive care to stabilize their bites and repair their teeth.

Now I'm one of the core faculty at the OBI Foundation and I've been on the Board of Directors for many years. Shortly after joining the board, we moved the teaching center to Denver and moved the office to a suite in my building in Missouri. Five years after moving the teaching center and administrative office to

Missouri, the OBI Foundation is thriving and solvent.

My life, after The Schuster Center Program, has been vastly different than it would have been. I am living my purpose, out front and out loud! I never missed a field trip or school performance with my kids. How amazing! I traveled the world, studying and vacationing, never worrying about my practice! I have three amazing children and have been married for almost 30 years. I really believe — none of this would have been possible without Dr. Schuster and the work I did with the Schuster Center. This work saves lives. This work enhances lives. This work impacts dentistry. This work preserves the highest level of caring in medicine. Without it — all we are left with is mediocrity.

## The Future

I meet with Dr. Schuster, other mentors, and OBI faculty regularly. Occasionally we discuss why dentists stay trapped in insurance-based, repair dentistry. I see it today all the time. Dentists keep taking clinical courses thinking, I'll just take another course because it's something I know. Here's what I do know so if I can learn more, then I can produce more.

But it's not true.

We don't know what we don't know. The difficulty is usually

a structural problem, and the structure is invisible. We can't see it because we're living in it. It's like counseling when they tell you something, and you think to yourself, how did I not see that? Well, you are in the structure or a pattern of behavior that's a subconscious loop. Patterns of behavior take away from what you want, but you don't know they exist. Those patterns can be mapped out, and there's always a thought or a belief behind all those patterns that can be discovered.

In 20018, I agreed to take on the CEO role of the Schuster Center and continue to grow the work of the Schuster Center, continue to improve the lives of dentists and physicians, preserve private care for patients, and preserve the legacy of Dr. Schuster and the Schuster Center.

I have devoted the rest of my career to helping dentists and physicians reach their full potential and live life "full out!" And it all starts with the work we do at The Schuster Center for professional development! I can't think of a better way to spend my life.

## About Dr. Michael Edwards, DMD, FABD

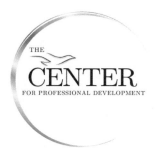

Dr. Edwards specializes in treating people with a unique, individualized approach, and has extensive training and experience to help even the most complex problems. Many patients are treated for symptoms but are never fully diagnosed, never to discover the root cause, or uncover patterns that led to the problem in the first place. Dr. Edwards focuses on providing a complete, thorough, comprehensive process that covers all areas of health to ensure his patients receive the care they are seeking.

Dr. Edwards is the CEO of The Center for Professional Development, and also serves as the President of the OBI Foundation for Bioesthetic Dentistry. Dr. Edwards teaches advanced dentistry as an OBI Core Faculty Member around the world, and regularly holds workshops based on his books: *Through the Red Sea, Are You Essential* and soon to be released, *The Heart of the Matter.* He is also the author of *The Cross of Life and Balancing Your Cross, as well as the creator of* the *Center's Time and Energy Planning System.*

## Dr. Edwards journey to The Center for Professional Development

"I was just ending my first year in private practice when I realized I was burned out. When my partner and I took over the practice of a retiring doctor, we simply continued the structures and systems already in place. It seemed to work. We kept the hours, the large team, all the marketing….

I was working 5 days a week with one late night, and every other Saturday. We were squeezing in 5-10 emergencies a day. Yes, we were making money, but I was working way too hard and would just sit at the end of the day and question — am I supposed to work like this for the next 40 years?

Once we entered the Center's Management Program, we immediately reduced our overhead and began changing the hours. As the overhead came down, we didn't need to work as hard. Not only did the pressure to produce come down, but we became more relaxed, and everything improved. We moved from a frenetic and stressed state to one focused on quality and getting to know people.

By the end of the year, our overhead was in model range — that means we went from an overhead in the high 70s to one in the low 50s. That equated to about 150-170K in additional profit, just from improving how the office operated.

I signed up for an additional two years of the Mastery Program (today this program is called "The Inner Circle" program) and not only got into the best shape of my life but ingrained the learning into the marrow of my being. I became a master at saving and investing, working with patients, and master planning, and began a CE path that has led me to teach at the highest levels of dentistry.

This is the type of program that has a Return On Investment (ROI) that can't be measured just in dollars. Because The Center is a school, you improve your systems and operations over time and it tends to get better as time goes on, increasing the ROI — year after year. But money isn't the only measure of ROI or success. What about our most precious resources? Our health. Our time. The team we work with — the people with whom we spend the most time!

This program is special and unlike any other in dentistry. Many places have tried to copy it over the years, but those copies are faded versions of what the program was and nowhere close to what it is today. The program continues to evolve with the times while maintaining the core principles of the learning.

Recent grads have reported a decrease in their overhead of 20-40%, increases in net profit that have more than doubled during their program, and in the case of a doctor 5 years out, profit increased from 39K to 400K. That is a nearly two million dollar swing in new money every five years all the while the doctor is doing the kind of work she loves doing!

My wish is to share it with as many of those seeking to practice a different way, to really enjoy the freedom of being a private care doctor, and to live a life in line with your deepest held values and beliefs."

**Dr. Edwards Contact information:**

michael.edwards@cfpd.com

Direct phone: 636.234.7481

Appointments with Dr. Edwards may be made using this link: https://bit.ly/edwardscalendar

# Chapter Fourteen
# Raymond Hsu, DDS, MAGD, LLSR
## Seattle, Washington

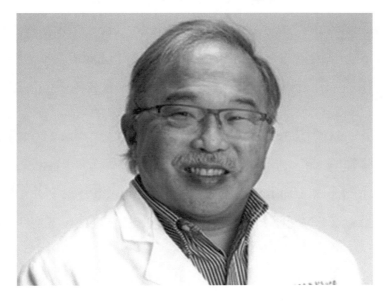

*Two strategies I learned from the Schuster Center were transformative.*

*These were the Dental Fitness Program and the concept of a written*

*Masterplan. These strategies were a win for patients and a win for our*

*office. They became key cornerstones of my practice.*

*For me, the Schuster Center was life changing.*

# The Nightmare

It's a bad memory from dark times eight years into my career. I was doing a recare exam for a young woman in hygiene. The hygienist told me the patient was flossing and had good home care. I looked at her red, swollen gums, and then I felt sick. The patient was coming in every six months for preventive care and her mouth looked sick. It's totally pointless I thought! I walked away thinking the patient was better off not seeing us if this was the result.

That experience and others like it had me close to selling my practice. Many of my patients worked at Microsoft where it was common to work 100 hours a week. I imagined that I would prefer the craziness of Microsoft, to being a dentist. How had I come to this?

# Following the Crowd

After graduating from the University of Washington dental school, I thought production was the measure of success in private practice. Like the first dentist I worked for, I wanted to build a monster practice, yet still do high-quality work. Isn't that the American Dream, "bigger is better?"

I dabbled with a few marketing schemes like a large ad in the yellow pages. I sought advice from dental consultants. I was driven by a passion for success. I started with two consultants who helped me get bigger and bigger. One consultant had me add assisted hygiene. A dental assistant helped the hygienist work out of two chairs (a profitable way to run hygiene, though not always appreciated by the patients.) Soon I had five operatories going at once. Three hygiene chairs were prebooked many weeks ahead. I was double booked with patients in two rooms. I maximized expanded duties for auxiliaries so I could delegate some procedures and see more patients. So what if ungrateful patients would cancel or not show up? My staff would fill those holes.

Production increased, but it was a challenge to keep pace with the schedule. My production numbers were outstanding! After six years, according to one dental journal, my production was in the top 5% of the nation. My dental colleagues in Seattle were blown away. I was averaging over 70-80 new patients a month, and I was taking home lots of money!

## Crisis—Personal Collapse as a Repair Factory Dentist

But there was a dark side. Occasionally at work, I had a tightening of my chest, and I had difficulty breathing. This was in the middle of seeing patients! How could that be? I was in my young thirties, trim, and physically active. When those gasps for air reverberated in my ears, the reality was I wanted to do something else. I hated being a dentist. I felt like a fraud, even though culture said I was a success. I needed to get out of dentistry before I killed myself.

I didn't understand why I had a high staff turnover. I was the one who was stressed.

Further, I was having problems at home. I could not understand my sudden, explosive fits of anger. It was scary for my beloved wife and scary to me. I was providing for my family, right? But it was the inability to breathe that finally got me. It felt like a heart attack. A psychologist friend with the same problem said I was having panic or anxiety attacks. It was common. That advice was a painful slap in the face. I realized that I wanted out of dentistry.

*Well, as Pogo would say, "We have met the enemy . . . and he is us."*

## Rescue

At that time, a local consultant introduced me to a management tape series by Dr. Michael Schuster. It made sense to me when he talked about slowing down, managing your money, and taking better care of your patients. "Slowing down" and "less is more" was revolutionary thinking! But it resonated with my core values, Matthew 15:15, and the Golden Rule. I scheduled time with an analyst to assess my practice. That was the start of my journey with Dr. Mike Schuster back in 1991. It inspired me to travel multiple times from Seattle to Scottsdale, AZ for classes. Travel for CE was something I never would have considered (or did) previously.

I found Mike Schuster to be a tough teacher. His intensity offended and scared some folks. They didn't see his intensity of caring. Despite his gruff exterior, I never met a man who cared for his fellow man so deeply.

It's a common human malady to wait and let the world come to you. Especially doctors who feel they've arrived after graduating from dental school. We aren't trained to manage a business. The apparent solution to problems is adding technology or the latest gizmo to produce more and make more money. We forget that there is a person attached to the teeth. To change direction, I felt like Sisyphus pushing the rock up that long, never-ending hill over and over again. A loving, firm tap to the back of the head from Mike Schuster was needed to wake me up and get me to make some changes.

He opened my eyes to another way; I began transforming the Hsu office. I wanted to care for patients more distinctively. I wanted to show them love. I wanted to replace high volume with high care

189

and quality. I saw the potential but there was a huge risk! In fact, it was downright scary. Not changing the practice would be a bigger risk, and maybe the death of me. I was damaged and spiraling downward. I needed to be vigorous and whole again. I had to find a better way for me. I felt like I was being ripped apart!

With the help and coaching of the Schuster Center, I mapped out a plan. The key to successful change was to identify my core values, picture my desired future, implement the strategies I was learning, and connect them together. I needed to hire employees who shared my values. I needed to attract the right patients. I let go of trying to keep every patient, and I focused on better serving those who were the right fit for our office.

## The Commitment

One of my core values is excellence, which requires persistent, ongoing learning. I aggressively pursued continuing education. In 1990, I received my Fellowship from the AGD, Mastership in 2000, and my LLSR (Lifetime Learning Service Recognition) in 2013. I'm proud of these credentials. However, I learned advanced clinical training is useless without communication skills to help patients want the treatment they need, innovative treatment, and long-term solutions.

Excellence demands focus. I revisited my mission statement from my early years as an associate. It still rang true. But now I actively use it as a filter for decision-making. Here was a dream that could come alive!

## Finding Magic—From Mechanic to Healer

Two strategies I learned from the Schuster Center were transformative. These were the Dental Fitness Program and the concept of a written Masterplan. These strategies were a win for patients and a win for our office. They became key cornerstones of my practice. Both systems are consistent with modern learning theory, engaging people in how they can help themselves, and helping people think long-term about their health. The Masterplan is where the patient's aspirations, hopes, and dreams for their health come to life. It's the essence of health care and the opposite of managing disease. Health is a notion of the future, and where you want to go.

Mike changed my thinking forever when he performed an oral exam on me during a workshop. I remember it vividly. At the end, he assessed my oral hygiene and used a black, gum stimulator to check for plaque on my teeth. I had no plaque and a 100% plaque-free score. But he brushed my teeth anyway to demonstrate proper technique. I realized I had never learned to brush correctly by reading from a book in dental school. I made a promise to myself at that time. I decided to brush the teeth of every new patient as Mike did for me. This is going to be the big reveal at the end of their exam—how to brush. I didn't know how to brush properly, and I know a lot of people out there who probably don't either.

Dental Fitness emphasizes education and prevention. This was the way! Patients got healthier and needed less patchwork repair. It reinforced my vision of helping people avoid dental treatment. We documented this with an in-office study of 105 patients followed over a ten-year period. It was proof of concept! Patients understood they were controlling the causes of disease, and not reacting to the damage after it occurred. Dr. Schuster taught us that what people want most is the least amount of dentistry. That resonated with me, and I took it to heart.

With the Masterplan system, my office attracted patients who were a good fit with our philosophy of health and comprehensive care. We didn't need to tell patients we were different or better. It was obvious by what we did.

*"Don't listen to what someone says they believe, just watch what they do." Dr. Schuster*

A doctor/patient relationship of trust is established at the first visit. This trust helps patients be more receptive to our recommendations. In time, they request comprehensive care and long-term solutions. With active disease under control, patients are confident to invest in lovely, long-term restorations for their health and smile. I'm able to utilize my advanced clinical training!

Something else I learned is to develop and invest in my staff. It's a huge benefit to have long-term staff that understand and support my philosophy of care. My profit-sharing plan includes employees. One hygienist was in the office for over 24 years, and she retired at age 66 with $400,000 (more in today's dollars if adjusted for inflation) in her account. She's grateful, and I'm happy I was able to help her achieve security for retirement.

## Legacy

I made exceptional progress during the Management year with the Schuster Center. So, I enrolled in the Mastery Program to continue working ON my practice and get closer to my vision. Eventually, that program was retitled Performance Coach, and for a while, I helped as a mentor for other dentists in the program.

Post Schuster Center I work less, but my production per hour increased so that I net more profit now than I did before. I trimmed off twelve days a year of work. I've gone from six employees to four and from fifty new patients a month to eight. My overhead dropped by tens of thousands of dollars after that first year. I work in two operatories rather than five. My office space has been downsized by about twenty percent. I have fewer headaches and annoyances to deal with. I still use the computerized Dental Fitness Program, and I've used digital radiography since '98. I have four articulators and I use all four constantly. I have a few dental toys, but technology is not the centerpiece of my practice. We focus on how we can help people get healthy, not fancy equipment for repair.

In the last two decades, I've had time to enrich my personal life. I started a Cub Scout pack and was the founding Cubmaster. I was the founding scoutmaster for a Boy Scout troop. I keep myself physically fit. I've been strong enough to hike three fifty-mile trips in the past six years. I've traveled the country, volunteered at a clinic for the disabled, and pursued a cappella barbershop singing as a hobby.

After thirty-five years I'm still married to my wonderful wife, who stood by me despite those early horrible years in practice. I saved enough to put three kids through college and let their mother stay home with them during their formative years. Despite some economic downturns I have achieved financial independence.

My workdays are more relaxed now. Instead of 30-40 patients, my hygienist and I see 16-24 patients per day. I have time to care for patients as individuals. I create a personal connection with each patient, instead of selling products—implants, fillings, and crowns. Our relationship is built on trust and collaboration rather than distrust and fear. People ask for the best care I can provide, and I don't pressure them with hard sell. It creates a bond of trust and respect that's therapeutic for them and therapeutic for me!

Financially, I could have retired at sixty-two with enough savings to support my lifestyle. I've stayed in practice because I love dentistry now. The practice has become like a hobby because I don't need the income. Recently, I reduced my workdays to half-time. I especially enjoy seeing friends who have been coming to the practice for decades. It's rewarding to be in their lives. I can't put a monetary value on that. I'm doing the dental procedures that I enjoy doing, and I work every day with a team of people I enjoy being with. Why would I give up my Dream Job?

What was the cost? I had to set aside time to put down the drill and work ON my practice. I had to take time to work on myself. I developed my people skills, leadership ability, and clinical skills. It took courage to be different from other dental offices, to break from insurance-driven, disease care, and to humble myself with mentors like Dr. Schuster. It was alarming when I dropped PPOs, and some patients left the practice. But it's rewarding when some of those same patients returned because they were disappointed elsewhere.

I slowed down and recovered my health and my patients got healthier. The chest pain and panic attacks are gone. I'm no longer buried in problems. The Schuster model changed my professional role from a tooth mechanic to a teacher, health coach, and physician of the mouth. I care for people, not just their teeth. I'm rewarded financially, emotionally, and with a life of purpose and passion.

The Schuster Center is inspiring. It lifts you up. I walked out after lectures inspired to be better, to grow. I'm so happy being a dentist now, and I wasn't back then. For me, the Schuster Center was life changing. I have a favorite quote from Calvin Coolidge that I like to share with friends, Scouts, and students.

*"Nothing in the world can take the place of persistence. Talent will not; nothing is more common than unsuccessful men with talent. Genius will not; unrewarded genius is almost a proverb. Education will not; the world is full of educated derelicts. Persistence and determination alone are omnipotent."*

*Raymond Hsu, D.D.S., MAGD, LLSR, practices Wellness Centered Dentistry in Redmond, WA, a suburb of Seattle. He graduated from the University of Washington Dental. He specializes in restorative dentistry, as well as treating conditions like sleep apnea and occlusal disease.*

*Dr. Hsu is a clinical instructor at the University of Washington School of Dentistry. He has taken over 2,000 hours of continuing education courses in all aspects of general dentistry, with a special emphasis on Bioesthetics. A crowning achievement was recognition by the Academy of General Dentistry, where he earned his fellowship and mastership, with its Lifelong Learning and Service Award in 2014. Dr. Hsu was only the 113th recipient of the commendation in the world.*

*Dr. Hsu enjoys hiking, golfing, reading, and singing with the Northwest Sound Chapter of the Barbershop Harmony Society.*

*Dr. Hsu and his daughter, Hannah, a research scientist, analyzed his patient data to study the effectiveness of the Dental Fitness Program. Dr. Hsu initiated the study after learning that one-third of general dentists do not regularly probe the periodontal pockets of their patients and that the average patient has a plaque-free score of only 49%. He monitored 105 patients with the Dental Fitness System over a ten-year period. All the patients in this group completed the preventive and corrective measures of their Masterplan. The average plaque-free score for this group was 88%. There were no teeth lost in this group. Of this group, 71% had no decay. Extrapolating data from the study shows that a patient who maintains a plaque-free score of 88% needed only 1.6 restorations for decay in a fifty-year period!*

*Learn more at*

https://www.wellnesscentereddentistry.com/page/meet-the-doctors/

# Chapter Fifteen
# Dr. TJ Bolt
## Omaha, Nebraska

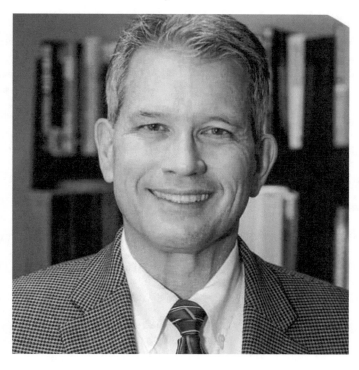

*My story is a journey towards mastery, to use my God-given talents to serve a purpose. I wanted to become the best I could be. Through study and self-discovery, I determined that I wanted to make a significant difference in the lives of my patients. I wanted to help people become as healthy as they chose to be. I wanted to be a dental health coach and help my patients prevent disease... Health-centered and Patient-centered care is the road less traveled. But it's the road with the biggest rewards. The rewards are not just making a living but making a difference. There is no other place in the world like the Schuster Center.*

## Start-Up Survival

After graduation in 1984, I bought a declining practice in Omaha, Nebraska. The owners had mismanaged it, and there were few remaining patients. I put profits back into the practice to keep it running, and my wife was able to support us. The third year was the turning point. I paid off the bank loan, and I could take a salary.

Early in my career, I was fearful of insurance companies controlling my destiny. A PPO insurance plan came out introducing the dental community to the first Managed Care Plan of Omaha. There was heavy pressure to accept a reduced fee schedule. Pandemonium and infighting broke out among dentists. We felt our livelihood was threatened, and we were all scared it would take patients from our practice. I never signed any insurance contracts. I formed a pact with some colleagues. We promised to hold each other accountable to never join managed cost plans. That pact is still in place thirty years later.

## Growth—Lost at Sea with Disease Care Mania

*"You don't need a relationship to treat someone's disease."*

With lots of hard work, I built a practice based on my paradigm from dental school—repair dentistry for patients with decay and gum disease. After ten years I had a busy practice, and I was earning a stable income. Then I completed coursework at the Pankey Institute. Pankey spoke of being a "physician of the mouth." I developed better clinical skills, and philosophy, and learned about the stomatognathic system. The practice generated profit, but I was NOT happy.

I felt like I was selling products. I was making money but making little difference in the health and lives of my patients. I was burned out and stressed about the future of my practice. I didn't understand why at the time, but I remember having a sick feeling on Wednesday and Sunday nights, about returning to work the next day. I was off on Wednesdays. A friend noted it was like having two Mondays in one week. It was a job, but why?

Fortunately, my attitude and abilities were about to change for the better.

## Finding Magic—A Wizard Appears and Shows a New Paradigm

Dr. Mike Schuster entered my life in 1987. I received his newsletter and heard him speak a few times. Seeds were planted, but the true meaning of his model didn't make sense yet.

Despite the Pankey instruction, I couldn't put the principles and methods into practice in a consistent manner. Pankey kept me in a high-volume model that was very stressful. What was missing became clear later. I finished up courses at Pankey and enrolled in the one-year Management Program at The Schuster Center for Professional Development.

In 1995 Mike Schuster invited dentists nationwide to attend a conference regarding the impact of insurance companies on dentistry. I was primed for action! I was concerned about the continued success of my practice, and I wanted my patients to understand that we were different. It turns out, that the Private Care Conference was a crucial experience in my practice career.

350 dentists from all over the United States came together for three days. We created the Private Care Creed. It means as much to me now as when we composed it. It's what I live by every day, and it continues to energize me.

The Management curriculum at The Center for Professional Development was fabulous. I still remember the excitement of learning how to create systems that put me in control of my practice for the first time in my life. I began to feel like the person God meant for me to be.

With these two experiences, the Private Care Conference and the Management Program at the Schuster Center, I was transformed! Now I had energy, excitement, and zeal. I found the purpose for why I was placed on the planet. The transformation put me on a lifelong journey that continues to energize and motivate me.

## Maturity—Sharing the Gift of Health Back Home

*Health is a function of collaborative relationship with each patient.*

After ten years of the proper coaching, and refining the right model, I have the practice of my Dreams. I help people break out of the disease cycle if they are sick, and I help them stay healthy. Further, I have a supportive, secure environment for my team. I love being a dentist and I love helping people in a significant way—to make a difference in the quality of their lives.

In summary, The Schuster Center transformed my practice AND my personal life.

- I learned how to control time and money for a better practice and life.

- I learned the art of the New Patient Examination, and how to fully engage patients.

- I learned that communication and leadership is an ongoing process of sustained study and practice—the process of mastery.

- I learned that I needed to spend time working ON my practice, and not just work IN the practice.

- I learned to appreciate that a full, interdependent relationship with my patients, my family, and my friends required me to work on myself. Indeed, I was surprised to discover this was the most important part of freedom from control by insurance companies.

- I learned that the right mentor/coach is key to the developmental process.

I continued to study at the Schuster Center after the Management course. I enrolled in a curriculum specific to behavioral growth called Mastery. Today the course is called Performance Coach. Behavioral study developed my people skills, in the office and in my personal life. I'm not just a better dentist. I'm a better spouse, a better parent, and a better friend.

We say at the Schuster Center "Structure influences behavior, but behavior determines results." It means creating a structure or a system to help people understand what is important to them. Then you become their advocate. They make better decisions for themselves and ask you for help (to do their dentistry).

That has been key to my fulfillment as a dentist. I just help people get what they want. I have become, through the guidance of the Schuster Center, a "Health Centered Dentist", and a "Success Planner". It's a transaction to treat a patient's disease. It becomes a transformation when I work together with each patient to prevent disease and create health. It's what was missing for me in the dark times of 1995.

*"The key in dentistry is personal relationships."*

Daily, I reconnect to what drew me to dentistry long ago—helping people and personal relationships. Now I can work in partnership with patients to help them attain something they couldn't do by themselves. It's priceless!

## Legacy

In conclusion, Health-Centered and Patient-Centered Care are the roads less traveled. But it is the road with the biggest rewards. The rewards are not just making a living but making a difference. There is no other place in the world like the Schuster Center.

I set aside a year of personal and practice expenses as a reserve or emergency fund. As I became financially secure, I've grown to regard patients differently. Patients don't feel rushed into treatment. They understand that I'm there to serve them at their own pace, not push them at my pace.

I organized my practice to foster interdependent relationships instead of co-dependent relationships. Mike Schuster helped me understand my role in that process. He helped me understand the Disease Cycle and how to help people get beyond the disease to have a more successful future. I learned that I need to study behavioral skills in addition to clinical dentistry.

Dr. Schuster helped me increase my self-esteem and my confidence to be a health advocate for my patients. He taught me to help people make good decisions for themselves, and in so doing accept higher levels of dental care.

I learned that patients are the only ones who have the power to create health. A doctor cannot give them health or cure them. Dental disease can't be cured but it can be controlled. This is why a partnership must be formed. I am now in the process of studying the connection between the mouth and the rest of the body (systemic).

The Schuster Center helped me slow my practice down. It allowed me to have time for my patients and my family, and to become optimally profitable. I learned how to inspire my team and my patients to make a difference in their lives. I focus on the dentistry I enjoy doing, and I market to the public appropriately. I attract patients who are looking for what I offer and what I enjoy doing. In other words, I have a clear purpose, and it's led to personal and professional fulfillment. I help people have the freedom, the power, and the opportunity to choose health.

*Dr. Thomas J. (TJ) Bolt graduated from Creighton University School of Dentistry. He opened his first dental practice in 1984. While developing his practice in Omaha he also worked as a part-time clinical instructor at the Creighton University School of Dentistry until 1994. He completed training at the LD Pankey Institute in Key Biscayne, Florida, and all the programs at The Schuster Center in Scottsdale, AZ.*

*Currently, he serves as a faculty member and a mentor for The Schuster Center and is a member of the American Dental Association, Omaha Executive Club, IAOMT, and the Academy of General Dentistry. He has served as past President of the NE Academy of General Dentistry, Omaha District Dental Society, Southwest Omaha Kiwanis, Omaha's Chamber of Commerce, President of the Development Committee for St. Vincent DePaul Church, President of the R.V. Tucker International Gold Study Club (since 1999).*

*https://drtjbolt.com/our-dental-team/*

# Chapter Sixteen
# Dr. Sharon Dickerson
## Denver, Colorado

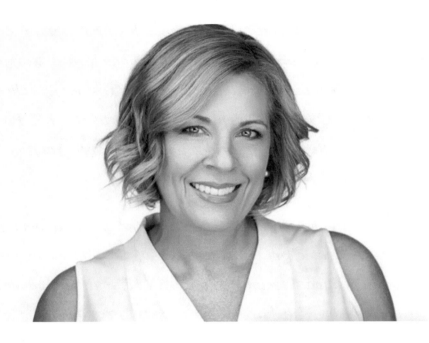

*I heard about the Schuster Center from my dear friend, Dr Tom Blake. In addition to financial struggles, I was having staff turmoil and some staff turnover. The practice was out of control. I called Tom in a panic mode. He said, "I've told you this Sharon, if I could come to Michigan and take your hand and walk you to Scottsdale, I would. You need to get to the Schuster Center." For me, the intangible benefits of living my dental life in my own way are the most important. I came to realize that it is very important for my professional expenditure of energy to be aligned with what I feel called to do.*

## Early Beginnings

I grew up in Battle Creek, Michigan, and I was involved in dentistry as a teenager. I was interested in science and medicine. My dad was a skilled general dentist, and I worked in his office during holidays and summers of high school and college. I helped with clinical assisting, administrative duties, and lab work. Prosthetics and restorative dentistry seemed artistic and creative. Also, I noticed my dad enjoyed close relationships with his loyal patients and their families.

During college, my dad told me to think about being a dentist. He said I had the hands for it. It seemed intimidating because there were few women dentist role models from my community at that time. I was privy to the business side of owning a practice by witnessing my father's ups and downs with the business. I remember a few times my dad and his partner had all their bills spread out on the desk wondering which ones they could delay paying, based on economic challenges.

After dental school, I became an associate in my dad's office. Early on, we worked out a buy/sell agreement, and over several years' time, I became the sole owner. I inherited financial systems in the practice (i.e. accounts receivable and accounts payable) managed by my mother and father with the guidance of their accounting firm. The practice produced well, but the nature of dentistry was changing when I took over. The cost of labor and technology was increasing, and in the absence of strategic planning, the practice was routinely struggling with cash flow.

My dad helped me begin learning about dental occlusion and complex restorative treatment. He encouraged me in my post-graduate training. Over several years I completed the curriculums of the LD Pankey Institute and The Dawson Center occlusal restorative programs. Gradually, my dad phased into retirement until he was working only one day a week. His production was good, but it was challenging for me to cover his part-time schedule. He would often complete a removable case, deliver the appliances, and then be out of the office for an extended period. I was charged with managing the post-operative follow-up and adjustments. It worked, but it became unwieldy and difficult to manage for me.

On the family front, I was under stress trying to navigate the natural flow of our family life with two young children. My husband worked full-time as a teacher, and our two children were in elementary school and daycare. Days often seemed chaotic, especially when one child was sick and had to be unexpectedly picked up from daycare in the middle of the day. There were no cell phones back then to sort things out, and I remember several times leaving a patient numb in the dental chair while I had to leave the office to pick up a sick kiddo. This was a conflict of interest for our family that was becoming increasingly untenable.

## Financial and Family Crisis

The practice hit a crisis about ten years after I took over. We were producing more than ever, but there wasn't enough cash flow to pay doctor salaries. Uncontrolled overhead was consuming doctors' compensation and profit. My dad offered to supply the practice a loan, with interest, to pay the doctor's salaries. I knew we were on a detrimental spiral, and my anxiety and uncertainty were at an all-time high. I knew my life and my practice were going in a direction that was not sustainable.

I'd heard about the Schuster Center from my good friend, Dr. Tom Blake. We had attended the Pankey Institute restorative program together. In addition to financial struggles, I was having staff turmoil and some staff turnover. The practice was, by all logical measures, out of control. I remember calling Tom in full panic mode. I didn't know what to do. He said, "I've told you this Sharon, and I'm going to tell you right now, if I could come to Michigan and take your hand and walk you to Scottsdale, I would. You need to get to the Schuster Center."

I took Dr. Blake's imperative to heart, and fortunately, I soon heard Dr. Mike Schuster's lecture at a one-day seminar in Lansing,

211

Michigan. He began by asking each dentist in the class to describe their practice situation. When it was my turn, I said I felt like I was out of my league, and I didn't know how to manage my practice. I mentioned my dad's continued but limited presence in the practice, and my feeling of inadequacy to navigate the business successfully.

Dr. Schuster asked me, "When is your father going to retire?" I answered, "I don't know, he hasn't said." I remember vividly what he said to me, in front of the entire class. "Well, that's something you need to figure out because you deserve to have a life as well." I hadn't ever thought of it this way, and it hit me like a ton of bricks. He was correct. I had the future of my practice and my family's welfare at stake. I simply had to figure this out.

At that time the practice had five days of hygiene per week and a staff of seven full-time employees. I was working four clinical days per week, and another full day for administrative tasks and lab work. Fortunately, based on my father's and my values, the practice was fee-for-service, and I had no contract or PPO plans. We processed insurance claim forms for patients, but we were under no insurance contracts.

I am forever grateful for this crisis, as it forced me to figure out how to add value to the patient care experience separate from their insurance limitations. In our manufacturing-centric town of

Battle Creek, Michigan, many of our patients had barriers to accepting dentistry that exceeded their annual policy maximums. These policy maximums had remained constant for many decades despite inflation. Additionally, we were constantly fighting against the insurance definitions of "reasonable and customary". Some ambiguous, faceless third party was interfering with my patient's dental care decisions, even though we weren't under any contracts. Managing a successful practice in this environment and helping patients to achieve and maintain long-term dental health became my primary priority.

## The Management Year

I followed up after that fateful seminar with a Practice Health Evaluation (PHE) by an analyst from the Schuster Center. He did a thorough financial assessment of the practice and interviewed the staff, my father, and me. Then he laid out the changes needed to reduce my stress and improve cash flow and profitability. He showed me the results of other dentists who had completed the one-year Management Program. He explained that getting organized with proper systems to control time and money would generate over $56,000 in additional profit. That profit would cover my tuition for the course, and then contribute to my income and wealth potential for every year after that.

I didn't know how I would follow through, but I felt my family and my career depended on it. Initially, my dad wasn't supportive, and I had to convince my husband to curtail his teaching career so that one of us was available to care for our young children. I truly give my husband credit for having the courage to make a tough decision for our family. He said, "We've got to have some assurance your practice is going to make it if I place my teaching career on hold. I'll become a stay-at-home dad if you agree to go through the Schuster Center and get control of the finances of the practice." This became our focus, and I committed to the Schuster program.

The Management year was intense because we added working ON the practice, learning new habits, and implementing systems. We had a two-hour staff meeting every week, which we had never done previously. I was writing up the assigned policies/systems late at night after the kids were asleep. We traveled as a staff to Scottsdale three times that year. I felt committed to doing the course exactly as it was laid out. I felt that my life and the welfare of my family depended on me doing the work in order to get the practice to a viable financial status.

My staff was hesitant at first. Gradually, I became clear about my vision for the practice, and I was able to articulate this in our developmental processes with The Schuster Center. I lost one valued staff member in this process, as she wouldn't align with my vision. While this was difficult, it was the right thing to do.

Fairly quickly, the staff realized that getting control of money and the daily schedule had real benefits for them. They could count on an actual lunch hour and go home on time at the end of the day. We reduced the daily chaos of treating emergency toothache patients who weren't in a mindset of long-term health. I came to accept that there are many other dentists who can service those patients. I was interested in partnering with patients who wanted to develop and maintain their health for their lifetimes. Percentage budgeting and regularly tracking key performance indicators helped us to create positive results very quickly. Within six months, the systems we created based on the Schuster Center training were having an immensely positive impact.

My new patient process had improved from my training at the Pankey Institute. But in my work on the New Patient Experience with Dr. Schuster, my skills became enhanced, and my results related to case acceptance improved dramatically. Dr. Mike Robichaux, a long-time mentor dentist at the Schuster Center, showed me how to make the Review of Findings consultation more visual so that patients had a better understanding of their problems. I also learned to contrast the visual picture of dental health vs. disease. While this may sound simple, I did not have the communication skills to accomplish this before my Schuster training. My coaches, mentor, and Dr. Schuster assisted my professional development very dramatically.

As I have continued to work with the principles, I found that I love the new patient process. I love helping patients understand the causes of disease. Once they understand their current reality and how they got to their current state, they are much more open to moving forward with comprehensive care. I've continued to refine and enhance the process every year since then.

## Performance Coach and a Niche Practice

I stayed connected to the Schuster Center after the Management Program in a program called Leadership. Now it's called Performance Coach, and I was a mentor for the first class of Performance Coach. The work that my colleagues and I did together in that program helped us to further define our values, become better leaders, and create a pathway in dentistry to fulfill our life purpose. I completed OBI, a multi-year program for advanced occlusal restorative dentistry. Further, I got seriously involved with holistic, or biologic dentistry.

The 2008-2009 economic downturn hit Michigan and the automotive industry quite hard. My financial advisors determined that the location of my practice was limiting my success. They encouraged me to move because other dentists with similar backgrounds and training in other parts of the country were having greater financial success. I was divorced by then and I was stalled with few personal or business prospects. In 2015, after much personal reflection with Dr. Schuster and his wife Patti, I sold my practice and moved to Denver, Colorado. Mike helped me find an associate position in an integrative dental practice that needed a biologically inclined dentist to handle complex restorative cases.

After a few years, I realized that I couldn't do what I felt called to do until I had my own practice again. Recently, I found the right space and built out a new office, specifically designed for my skills, interest, and the patients that come to see me. Its 1900 square feet, with three treatment rooms, and a spacious consult room. I built out the space from scratch in 2019 and opened a brand-new practice based on my values and priorities. My office space and practice are perfect for what I want to do now.

Here's the fascinating thing about my startup. It's not easy to get financing for the buildout and all the necessary equipment in the later stages of a career. I needed $500,000 to get the practice started. My financing was rejected by several banks. Ultimately, I was given a chance by Wells Fargo. They had serious questions, and I remember making a PowerPoint presentation to the dental financing board to justify my startup practice. I had to explain how

I planned to be successful as a dentist in such a competitive market without accepting insurance plans. So, I showed them what I had already done in Michigan, and how I had made professional connections in Denver. They took a chance and gave me the loan. I could not have managed that process without my business understanding from the Schuster Center.

## Benefits

For me, the intangible benefits of living my dental life in my own way are the most important. I came to realize that it is very important for my professional expenditure of energy to be in alignment with what I feel called to do, and with what I feel my creator has set me here to do.

If I were in the world of traditional dentistry, without influence from the Schuster Center, I feel like I'd be in a state of dissonance. I truly don't think that I would be healthy or happy. It would be emotional, and I don't think I could be physically and mentally healthy if I was at odds with how I really want to be with people, with my patients, and with my staff.

Of course, the tangible benefits are significant. I'm really, grateful to have a model of practice that works, to have a basic business acumen, and to know how to control a business budget and a well-organized patient schedule. I sincerely appreciate knowing the basics of how to control my time and cash flow so that I can organize a business model around that. I have objective criteria for my decisions which is a big confidence builder. I can manage my staff, my bills, my marketing, and everything I spend in the practice based on data analysis and foundational values.

My current practice is fee-for-service. I don't submit insurance forms for patients anymore. This isn't because I don't want to help them, but because the engagement with dental insurance acts as a distraction from what my patients and I decide is most important in our work together. Patients come to my office from various parts of the state and the country. I see three new patients per week and commit two full hours of my time with them at that initial visit. I use block scheduling, and I don't have a hygienist in the office currently. Patients come in for treatment, complete their treatment, and then have their periodontal health maintained elsewhere by their general dentist. They come back for an annual exam and any necessary maintenance of their dental restoration. I believe in the importance of the dental hygiene department and am comfortable with what I'm seeing in terms of my patient's periodontal health over time with their local dental practices.

My career path has had some dramatic ups and downs. I have been blessed with many important mentors that have helped me to forge a positive pathway. I feel grateful for the influence of Dr. Schuster and the entire staff over the years at The Schuster Center for being such an important influence on me having a productive, fulfilling life in dentistry. It's an awesome profession that allows dentists to form profound relationships with their patients and offer treatment that can truly enhance people's longevity and quality of life. We have the option to be business owners and thereby express ourselves at all levels through the organization. I'm very glad that my father encouraged me to become a dentist all those years ago.

*Dr. Sharon Dickerson has a holistic and biological dental practice in Denver, CO. She offers advanced restorative dental techniques with the principles of biological dentistry for dynamic, long-term dental solutions. Dr. Dickerson has an extensive background in occlusal restorative dentistry, including Pankey, Dawson, and Orthognathic Bioesthetics (OBI). She remains active in OBI, currently serving on the Board of Directors for the organization. She has been a member of the IAOMT (International Academy of Oral Medicine and Toxicology) since 2003 and is committed to mercury-safe practices. She also implements her training in the use of oxygen/ozone treatments as it pertains to optimum dental procedure outcomes. Learn more at https://sharondickersondds.com/about-us*

# Chapter Seventeen
# Dr. Fred Arnold
## Traverse City, Michigan

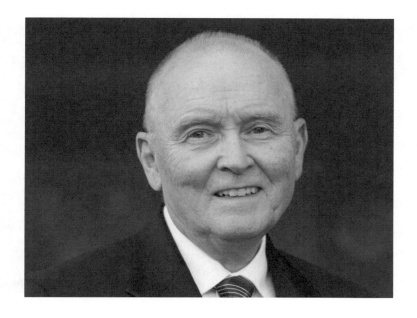

*Dr. Schuster's integrity and patient-first attitude got my attention. The strategies he taught were congruent with my professional values. His respect for patients was a game-changer. He said, "Less is more." That's what I was looking for.*

## The Early Years

After dental school, I gained a range of clinical experience with two years in the Air Force. One experience was a premonition of ethical decisions to come in private practice. The AF clinic was an open door, and I was watching a contest between two dentists. They were racing to see who could prep and fill a DO amalgam the fastest. The record was two minutes and 21 seconds. I didn't think it through at the time, but that struck me as wrong. Was speed the goal? What about quality? Why not the best instead of the fastest?

I started private practice with a small office in Traverse City, MI, and a single dental assistant. A year later I merged with the established family practice of Dr. Chuck Kelly. Chuck was my first mentor. He was clinically skilled, charismatic, honest, and a savvy businessman. He was a devotee of Dr. Robert Barkley, and he developed a full preventive program for adults and children. Further, Chuck was a student of behavioral psychology. He influenced me to study how people make decisions, and what motivates behavior. I learned that I needed to treat and trust the staff with the same respect that I did our patients.

Chuck and I attended many clinical and behavioral courses, but we often failed to implement what we learned. The staff patiently tolerated our post-lecture enthusiasm about changing office protocols. They had seen it before. In two weeks, the office routine would go back to normal.

A few years after merging my practice with Chuck's a problem surfaced. I had just presented and closed a full mouth restoration case. The problem was I had to explain to the patient I didn't know how to do that. So, I referred the patient to my qualified partner for the treatment.

It left me disappointed and frustrated. I'd just closed a big case, and I couldn't deliver the care! What was I thinking? I immediately called the Pankey Institute. I described my situation to Dr. Pankey's secretary, and she asked me to hold. Two minutes later Dr. Pankey came to the phone. "Hello, this is Dr. Pankey. Young man, I understand you have a problem. How may I help?" He invited me to Miami, Florida for classes. I enrolled to begin in three months. That decision gave me believable hope. I learned it's critical to step up and say YES to important things in life.

My practice grew as did my clinical skills. Then, another crisis occurred. With my Pankey training, I had become more skillful at diagnosing bite problems, or occlusal disease. Now I recognized patients with obvious occlusal interferences, abnormal wear, and a history of cracking and breaking teeth. These patients needed bite balancing (occlusal equilibration) to control damaging forces. However, Delta Dental would only approve equilibration for patients with periodontal disease. Many patients did not fit Delta's criteria, i.e., they had occlusal problems, but they had healthy gums. I struggled to figure out a way to bill the insurance for necessary corrective treatment.

## Drawing a Line in the Sand

Then the decision became clear. It was time to take a stand! I wasn't going to fudge my clinical findings to get treatment approved. Neither would I allow an insurance clerk to dictate how to care for my patients. I decided to drop participation with insurance companies and their treatment restrictions. When we described the situation to our patients one at a time most understood. Also, we learned that patients received reimbursement faster directly than our office did. Yes, some patients left our office. Fortunately, we offered enough added value that 90% stayed with us and embraced the new reimbursement process. The problem continues in dentistry to this day. How do third parties affect a dental practice, and the doctor's treatment recommendations? How do they limit doctor and patient choices? How can the doctor's service be worth more than the insurance company will pay?

## Growth and Disappointment

Eventually, I decided to establish my own practice separate

from the charismatic Chuck Kelly. The practice continued to grow with lots of children, parents, and grandparents. By 1989 I had a staff of seven with two hygienists, but I was increasingly unhappy getting bigger. The growth had exposed my weakness as a manager. Also, checking twelve to fourteen hygiene patients a day was disruptive. My focus would break, and it damaged my relationship with patients.

I remember an article in Dental Management Magazine describing the first Million Dollar Practice. I needed to do more procedures for more people if I was to reach that coveted goal. Success was defined by the dollar sign.

It was time for more help. I researched various dental consultants. I listened to Jim Pride of the Pride Institute. One memorable statistic showed that mid-career many successful dentists decide to build bigger and fancier buildings and add more staff. Unfortunately, most of those dentists were never as successful again, and never as happy as before. The new debt was a big setback. They needed more income, so they worked longer hours, hired more staff, saw more patients, and did more procedures. Exactly what I wanted to avoid! Indeed, I wanted to get smaller. I listened to the gurus who promoted "bigger and more" and became disillusioned.

Then I heard Dr. Michael Schuster speak at the Michigan

Dental Association meeting. He was an instructor at the Pankey Institute, then later opened a business school for dentists. His integrity and patient-first attitude got my attention. The strategies he taught were congruent with my professional values. His respect for patients was a game-changer. He said, "Less is more." That's what I was looking for.

An analyst from the Schuster Center spent two days evaluating my practice. He interviewed me and all the staff. He looked at our numbers and carefully listened to my goals. Two weeks later he reviewed his findings and analysis. He explained how implementing the Schuster model would improve our business practices, improve patient satisfaction, and reduce my time in the office by decreasing overhead and increasing my hourly production. My wife, Sue, was reluctant to enroll at first. She had seen me take too many classes and not make real progress. I was a chronic procrastinator. But after listening to the Schuster analyst she said, "You've got to do this!" She wrote the check and sent it in.

## On to Arizona – Discovering Magic

We began the Management Program at the Schuster Center. My core office team flew to Scottsdale—my office manager, my hygienist, my wife, and me.

Initially, we focused on getting control of time and money.

It started with two questions:

1.  How much is enough? If I don't know, then I'll never know how much is enough?

2.  What do I believe in? It went to the heart of my standards for patient care, staff relationships, and how to live my life. If I don't know my beliefs, then how will I ever measure success?

We learned about policies and systems (P&S.) P&S is the operating manual that guides everything we do, from answering the phone to financial arrangements to instrument sterilization. P&S would serve as our guide to get time and money under control. We started with twenty important ones. I started to gain control of my practice, and my life.

We set up twice-monthly phone calls with a coach from the SC to review key performance indicators (KPIs) and monitor our progress. Two staff members quit the first month. They didn't want to change. They were good people and I wished them well, but they weren't the right fit for my practice. Our goals and aspirations didn't match up. Retaining staff who don't support your mission results in poor performance, patient dissatisfaction, and an unhappy team. It stymies their satisfaction and practice growth.

That year my team and I made two more trips to AZ, and I made one by myself. These training sessions were called "Intensives." Each one was two and a half days of concentrated lectures, workshops, and team discussions. It was a serious process of growth.

- I learned how to introduce people to the practice and how to ask for referrals.

- The new patient process expanded to include an insightful interview with the patient prior to the oral examination. "Knowing your patient is more important than knowing their disease," took on new meaning. We learned how to engage new patients in their health, and how to listen carefully to their concerns.

- We monitored KPIs like production, collections, expenses, profit, new patients, case acceptance, and more.

- Case acceptance improved. The team and I enjoyed our time with patients more and more. Getting to really know someone is much more satisfying than racing to get a filling done in 2-1/2 minutes.

- We learned about job descriptions. We studied the books of the best minds in business and psychology. After the first twenty, we developed more policies and systems to govern operations and empower the team to manage the practice according to our shared vision. The team got energized and more efficient as their role in managing the practice increased, and they saw the practice improving.

- The future we hoped for was coming to life! Expenses and overhead were reduced, and profit increased, reflecting the impact of our P&S.

I made the difficult decision to stop seeing children. I enjoyed treating children, but that part of my practice was consuming too much time and energy. My clinical skills improved from training at Pankey and Advanced Restorative Seminars. I was equipped to handle the complex restorative needs of adults. Also, my improved communication skills prompted more patients to accept comprehensive treatment. I was seeing fewer patients, but I was taking better care of them.

Three years later, my hygienist reminded me where we had been. "When you stopped seeing children, we lost 40% of our patient base (400 active patients.) Some of their parents and grandparents left too. Yet, you are successful, and you are doing what you wanted." It's true. I went from more to less. But...

- I had two fewer employees, requiring less time for

management.

- I went from seven days of hygiene (and hygiene exam interruptions) to four days.

- I had more time off and my net profit was better than before.

- I eliminated anxiety and energy drain from treating children.

- I achieved my goals to control time and reduce office hours.

The bold belief that I could limit my practice to adults and still thrive occurred only because I applied the principles of the Schuster Center and they worked!

With practice operations and my personal time under control, we shifted emphasis to helping patients get healthy and making a significant difference in their lives. We adopted the Dental Fitness Program, which takes patients through the process of controlling infection and gum disease. Dental Fitness taught us the behavioral process of how people learn. The key was first engaging the patient in a trusting relationship. My hygienist resisted at first, but then she learned of the results obtained in four other offices using Dental Fitness. They loved it and reported an overall improvement in their patient's health. Many formerly resistant patients were now brushing and flossing regularly.

Three months later Michelle cornered me in the office. She said, "Do you know what my job is as an RDH? I finally figured it out! I am an educator, a communicator." She got it and so did our patients. One patient confided in Michelle "Wow, I've got to thank you! My wife hasn't kissed me like that in years!" We don't often get a chance to know how much we positively affect people's lives. Consider how periodontal disease affects other chronic inflammatory diseases such as vascular disease and diabetes. We can help people make marked improvements in their general health. I came into this profession to help people. Dental Fitness is the best tool I have found to do that. Period.

The last session in AZ was only for doctors. My takeaway was that humans are designed to grow in knowledge, experience, and relationships. When we stop growing in these areas we start to die. As we learn, we experience more joy in our relationships with our patients, our team, and above all, our families, and our God. I'll never regret the opportunity I had to say yes. Yes, to my wife, yes to Dr. Schuster, and yes to the rest of my life.

## Giving Back

My practice thrived after completing that year of study in 1992. Even more improvements occurred. I learned more about the biology of the oral facial system and how to restore and enhance its function and beauty. I engaged with the SC again in 1995 for a 2-year study program called Mastery. Seven of us studied together to build patient-centered and health-centered practices. It's critical to pursue personal growth if we want to practice outside insurance-driven care. A fee-for-service practice requires the ability to form trusting relationships. It's particularly true for patients needing extensive and expensive dentistry.

After Mastery I was invited to join the Center team as a mentor. Working with dentists focused on their personal, family, and practice growth has been an incredible experience for me. I am grateful for the opportunity to work with those professionals, and I feel I learned as much or more than they did. Many lifelong friendships were established in those groups.

In 2009 Mike started a program called Performance Coach. I mentored a group of 7 doctors for three years, growing, learning, and laughing together. We learned to trust one another, to share our stories, and to listen to others without judgment. That experience opened me to the world of truth. If we don't know what's true, or current reality, how are we to proceed with our lives and our practices?

We also had the opportunity to learn from renowned authors in business and psychology, including George Land, James Hollis,

Robert Fritz, and Jacob Needleman. We had the rare opportunity to form a Mastermind group. Thinking and laughing together we found solutions to some of our most vexing questions.

## Current Reality - 2015

I sit here looking out over the lake realizing that I have come home. I started out wanting to help others through my hands and my heart. I want to help those dentists who want to use their hands and hearts, their desire, and their growth to help their patients, teams, and their families towards a richer, healthier life. It starts with a "yes" and is followed with lots of work.

When you are ready to give the Schuster Center a call, ask for Dr. Schuster. He will come to the phone and intone those same words I heard so many years ago from Dr. Pankey, "Young woman, young man, I understand you want to talk. How may I help?" All you need to do is say yes.

# Chapter Eighteen
# Dr. Mary Isaacs
## Winter Springs, Florida

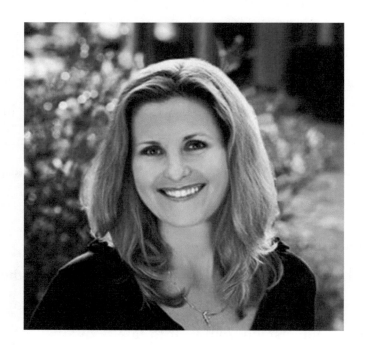

*I wasn't comfortable working in the production model of dentistry, jumping from room to room, and from patient to patient, trying to be efficient and maximize procedures. One of my core values is respect, and I felt like I was disrespecting the whole situation. It was stressful and frustrating. Dr. Schuster showed me a better way.*

*Dr. Schuster taught me a better practice model and how to develop deeper relationships with people. If I hadn't learned that I would never have been able to do the level of dentistry that I do today.*

# Why Become a Dentist?

I grew up with a gap between my front teeth. I was self-conscious about my appearance and didn't smile much. Then in the sixth grade, I got braces, and it really helped my self-esteem. That's when I became interested in dentistry as a career. I wanted to help other people have a confident smile, and I enjoy using my right brain, and creative side to recreate natural beauty and healthy function. Also, I wanted to be a professional and own my own business. My dad owned his own business and retired at age fifty-five. He encouraged me to do whatever I wanted, but he said, "Whatever you do, be the best."

I graduated third in my high school class. Few women went into dentistry in the 70s, so my guidance counselor recommended I go into dental hygiene. I worked as a hygienist for three years, and then my dentist employer, a woman, encouraged me to go to dental school. First, I completed dental school prerequisites (organic chemistry and physics.) My dental school class was about twenty percent women and I graduated sixth in the class. Then I did a one-year advanced education in general practice residency in Kansas City, Missouri. I started as an associate in the same practice where I'd been a hygienist. The owner gave me fifty patients and I worked out of one operatory. I worked long hours, five days a week, including some nights and Saturdays to build my practice.

After two and a half years I had enough patients to buy into the goodwill of the practice and half the equipment. We had two separate practices in a space-sharing arrangement. Our patient base grew larger, and we did an office buildout from five operatories to eight. We had three hygiene ops, two ops for each dentist, and one overflow operatory.

## Building Clinical Skills and Frustration with the Wrong Practice Structure

At first, I worked according to a production model popular with many consultants. Doctor and assistant time are scheduled in the appointment book for maximum efficiency and production. The goal is for the dentist to generate billable procedures and delegate reversible procedures to auxiliaries. For example, I would start a new patient exam. Then, while the assistant took radiographs, I would leave the new patient to place a crown on a different patient or check a hygiene patient. I wasn't comfortable doing that, and it felt like the patient wanted me to stay with them. One of my core values is respect, and I felt like I was disrespecting the whole situation. I found it stressful and frustrating.

I started taking courses at Spear in Seattle in 2004, and eventually, I took all the restorative courses they offered. I learned excellent techniques and improved my clinical skills. Spear used to have live courses where you flew your patient to Seattle and performed restorative treatment under faculty supervision. I did a live course in anterior esthetic dentistry. Dr. Bob Winter had me do three sets of veneers for my patient, and I tried them all in. It was a wonderful teaching moment for me.

After some years, I recognized I had the skills to deliver better dentistry than patients routinely accepted. The doctor I shared space with was still following the production model. In the morning huddle, we determined the monetary value of each patient according to the treatment they needed. It felt like patients had a dollar sign stamped on their foreheads. That bothered me. I thought, they were not a dollar amount, they were a person.

After fifteen years, the other dentist wanted to leave for mission work, so I bought her practice. I was already busy, and it wasn't my best decision. But I thought bigger would be better. The high-volume model was so engrained in my psyche that I didn't think clearly about what I really wanted for my practice. I didn't realize that I was getting even deeper into the wrong mode of practice—high volume, repair dentistry. Comprehensive patient care requires a strong doctor-patient relationship, not hopping from room to room to maximize efficiency.

## Change Begins with the Right Practice Structure —
## The Schuster Center Model

Around that time, I heard Dr. Schuster lecture at a Seattle Study Club meeting. He advocated a different model, doing more complete care for fewer patients, where high value is placed on the doctor-patient relationship. That connected with me. Everything he talked about was right for me. You've heard the saying, "When the student is ready, the teacher will appear." I realized I didn't need to run around like my head was cut off. On a readiness scale of 1 to 10, where one is not interested and 10 is super ready, I was a nine!

I enrolled in the Schuster Management Program. We started with a Practice Health Evaluation (PHE). I learned our production was good, but my overhead was high. So going into the Management year I had the following goals:

- I wanted to reduce my overhead from 70% and increase profitability.

- I wanted to get control of time and decrease stress from working long hours and jumping between multiple patients during the day.

- I wanted to implement my improved clinical skills and increase patient acceptance for more complete care— quadrant dentistry and full mouth dentistry.

238

I flew the staff out to Scottsdale, AZ with me three times over the year. At that time, I had two full-time hygienists, two front desk coordinators, and two dental assistants. One three-day session was memorable. My two chairside assistants were causing trouble, actively resisting change, and sabotaging my leadership. Their negativity infected the other staff members. With coaching from Dr. Schuster, and Brenda, the CFO of the Schuster Center, I fired the two assistants while we were in Arizona. It was traumatic but necessary. I told them they didn't fit with my practice philosophy and my core values. In retrospect, I should have fired them sooner. One assistant understood and accepted my decision. She even called me two years later to apologize for her poor behavior.

We returned to Florida that weekend. I had no chairside assistant on Monday. My receptionist helped me, and we made it work. Soon after I hired two amazing assistants and staff morale had a big boost. I told myself that would never happen again, and it hasn't. Except for that incident, my team dynamics have always been pretty good. I don't hire people who don't fit my philosophy and core values. I provide staff with good training, and I'm sensitive to staff issues having experience as a staff member myself for three years. One hygienist has been with me for twenty-six years, and she recently received myofunctional training to coach patients for better breathing.

### The Right New Patient Process Transforms My Practice

My favorite part of the Management Program at the Schuster Center was reducing practice overhead and improving my new patient process. I learned to conduct an open interview with the patient and not come in with an agenda. I learned to be a better listener and ask the right questions. In the past, I would have done the exam and the treatment plan at the same time. Now I start where the patient is at, find out what they want, and guide them where they want to go. I educate them and create tension by demonstrating where they are now and where they want to be. That tension pulls them toward their preferred future. It's significantly different than me pushing treatment on them.

I'm wrong sometimes, and then I need to go back to the beginning and figure out what the patient really wants. Sometimes patients want less treatment than I recommend and sometimes they want more than I initially think they will accept.

Now I love the new patient process. I get lots of background information ahead of time with a phone consult. When the patient comes in, we sit down for a one-to-one interview. My assistant is in the room to take notes, and we videotape the conversation. It's a big help to go back later and watch myself on video. I've learned a ton! I saw that I was doing all the talking and I needed to be a better listener. We do photography, blow up the photos on screen, and look at them with the patient. We see so many things, especially growth patterns with children, that we didn't see before.

One new patient experience is memorable. I'd done the exam a few days earlier, and her husband came in with her for the review of findings consultation. The three of us were looking at her intraoral and facial photos and she said, "I didn't realize my mouth was so bad, it's so ugly."

Then her husband said, "Honey, I had no idea. We should have done something sooner."

She was worried about the money, and that the cost would be too high. But he said, "No, we should take care of this." He loved her so much that he felt the cost was worth it. We did all her treatment, and the result was beautiful. She even did some promotion for me in a magazine with before and after photos.

The new patient process is critical, and it begins with the interview. I find out where they are, where they want to go, and how they think they will get there. I ask how it will make them feel if they get what they want, and how they will feel if they don't get what they want. I try to keep money out of the equation and find out what the patient really wants without considering the cost. That's important when learning their vision and expectations.

Then I do the clinical exam and the assistant takes radiographs. Depending on what I find clinically determines where we go next. Treatment plans can get involved and we take it one step at a time. We've gone beyond treatment solely for decay or gum disease.

## Saving Lives with Dental Sleep Medicine

I have a diploma in Dental Sleep Medicine, so we do a lot to address sleep problems in the practice. I got interested in sleep problems because my husband had six heart stents placed at age forty-five. He couldn't wear a CPAP. He's 62 now.

I started out doing appliances for mandibular advancement, but that can cause problems like bite opening. Now we use a multi-faceted approach to improve a poor airway. It can involve craniofacial development to widen the dental arches, myofunctional therapy, aligner therapy, and restorative treatment to stabilize the jaw joints and the bite, or any combination of all of the above.

Complex sleep and restorative cases with multiple treatment modalities require multiple reviews of findings and consultations along the way. The sequence is:

- First, control sleep and a normal airway.
- Second, stabilize the jaw joints/address TMJ issues.

- Finally, restorative treatment is needed to stabilize the bite and protect teeth. This can mean additive composite (especially for children and adults with virgin teeth), porcelain restorations, or a combination of the two.

Some patients don't follow through with treatment and that's OK. But they need to understand the consequences of not treating sleep apnea, and bigger things can happen down the road, like Alzheimer's or cardiovascular disease.

I like Vivos/craniofacial development therapy because it addresses the root cause of a poor airway, not just symptoms. It widens the dental arches and opens the airway and the nasal passages. TMJ patients are typically the sleep patients, they are the same person. It's rare that I see a TMJ patient who doesn't have sleep apnea.

Patients who follow through with treatment receive excellent value. Often, they no longer need to wear a CPAP, TMD is controlled, and they get back good function and esthetics. I think that covers all the bases.

Of course, I collaborate closely with their physician to get a sleep study and make a diagnosis before I recommend any treatment. Further, I need to know what medication the patient is taking and if they are on a CPAP. I send the written Review of

Findings from my clinical exam to the patient's MD. It's a medical document, so they need to read it. I ask the physician what they want to do, and I give them the patient's treatment preferences. Sometimes the physician misses the sleep apnea. Often, they say, "Who is this dentist?" They are amazed that I'm so thorough, and that I document all my findings for the patient in a report. Many physicians will contact me, refer patients to me, or become patients in the practice.

My husband's cardiologist became a patient in my practice. His mom had periodontal disease, and he understood the perio-cardiac link of the disease. He wanted to avoid periodontal disease and he came to us for saliva testing for HR5 and red complex of bacteria.

*Now I've become part of the Integrative Medicine team!*

It's incredible how the new patient system works. It's low-cost, internal marketing that attracts precisely the kind of patients my training has prepared me to help, and the patients I most enjoy helping. However, the final treatment plan is always the patient's decision. Usually, they have three or four options. They can choose surgery, craniofacial development, aligners, a CPAP, restorative treatment with composite addition or with porcelain, or some combination thereof.

# Long-Term Benefits of the Schuster Model

The Schuster model gave me structure and systems for relationship-centered, health-centered dentistry. Mike Schuster and the Center staff gave me and my team better verbal skills, listening skills, and a slower pace in the office for effective communication with patients. We do more complete care for fewer people who have high value for health, and who appreciate the personalized care we provide. My tagline is:

*Exceptional smiles for health. For life. Saving lives with complete care.*

After the Management Program, I stayed connected to the Schuster Center with the Performance Coach (PC) program. I recognized the power of coaching early in my career. I only know what I know. So, with my practice I have people looking at it from the outside. They help me be objective, discover new solutions, and make good decisions.

I was unconsciously incompetent after dental school. I didn't even know how much I didn't know. Then I became consciously incompetent, and I realized I needed more clinical training. I flew to Seattle from Florida and took all the clinical dentistry courses offered by Spear. I flew to Texas and took the year-and-a-half program at the Texas Center for Occlusal Studies run by Hal

Stewart. I completed training in Dental Sleep Medicine and aligner therapy. I completed craniofacial development training with Vivos. Now for most dentistry, I'm unconsciously competent. I know what to do without consulting an outside expert. There is always somebody better than me. I continue to learn from mentors in PC.

It always goes back to basics. For example, it's critical to have the right new patient process and to develop deeper relationships with people. If I hadn't learned that from the Schuster Center, I would never be able to do the level of dentistry that I do today. Dr. Schuster taught me a patient-centered, health-centered model of practice. It's rooted in a philosophy of patient care handed down by giants in dentistry like Bob Barkley, LD Pankey, and Harold Wirth. The Schuster Center helped me develop systems and practice structures so that patients want the treatment they need. We call that "getting what I've learned off the shelf." It includes acceptance for sleep dentistry, TMD therapy, preventive periodontics, and full-mouth restorative dentistry.

If I do what I'm supposed to do during the new patient exam and the Review of Findings consult, then my numbers are always in line. Profitability and case acceptance flow from that. It's never not there. So yes, we monitor practice numbers, but our energy isn't going in that direction, or into daily production goals. Rather our energy goes into the new patient process, building relationships, and providing health-centered treatment.

## Good Coaching and Partnering with Like-Minded Colleagues

With Performance Coach (PC) I'm in a group of like-minded dentists. They are a fantastic resource. We know each other and talk to each other every two weeks. I'm way closer to them than anyone in my local dental society. Colleagues in PC helped me pursue training in advanced restorative dentistry and Dental Sleep Medicine. One thing leads to another, and that leads to another. I call those God moments.

We help each other see things objectively and set goals. I like friends holding me accountable to accomplish my goals. It's like working with my personal trainer. He pushes me and gives me ideas way more than I can do myself. He monitors my weight and waist size and tracks my progress. It's the same with PC. We go over our numbers together to make sure we are following the Schuster Center model. Are we doing what we said we wanted to do? If I don't look at that then I don't know where my practice is. Occasionally, my numbers are off, but I understand why they're off, and then I'm okay with it.

Today, I'm doing exactly the kind of dentistry I want to do, and at a comfortable pace. I have less stress, and my profit has increased. Our overhead has decreased from 70% to 55%. I work four days a week, and I take off four weeks/year. I'm planning to go to three workdays/week this year. We limit new patients to 3-4/week. We have a two-hour staff meeting monthly. We do staff training, discuss any problems, and how to incorporate new technology. Both doctors work M-Th, 8-5. Each morning we have a huddle, and it starts with a leadership statement. Then we review all charts, patient preferences, lab cases, etc. so the day runs smoothly.

Most new patients have sleep problems or want full mouth restorative treatment, and all are referrals from existing patients or medical/dental specialists. My practice is getting so sleep-focused that I need to hire an associate dentist to handle some of the restorative treatment and to watch the office when I'm out. We get along well and share similar values.

I've never taken dental capitation or PPO plans. We accept dental insurance, and we file claims for patients, but my fees are not dictated by an insurance company. We don't get complaints from patients about how we handle insurance.

I've been teaching part-time at Spear in Scottsdale, AZ for fifteen years. When I retire, I want to leave a legacy and keep the practice going. I know we've built something special for patients and the dental team. I don't want all the hard work I've done over the years to get trashed by corporate dentistry that prioritizes business over patient care. I'm teaching my associate how to lead a patient-centered practice, and she's the most likely one to take over at some point.

*Dr. Mary Isaacs practices in Winter Springs, FL. She graduated from the University of Florida College of Dentistry with Honors and completed a one-year Advanced Education in General Dentistry Residency program at the University of Missouri in Kansas City.*

*Dr. Isaacs has received numerous awards, including the Academy of General Dentistry Achievement Award, the Quintessence Award for Clinical Achievement in Restorative Dentistry, the American Society of Dentistry for Children Merit Award, the American Association of Women Dentists Certificate of Recognition for Outstanding Leadership and Academic Excellence, and induction into Omicron Kappa Upsilon Honorary Dental Society.*

*She is a member of the American Dental Association, Florida Dental Association, Central Florida Dental Association, the Dental Society of Greater Orlando, Academy of General*

*Dentistry, Florida Academy of Cosmetic Dentistry, American Academy of Dental Sleep Medicine, Seattle Dental Study Club, Central Florida Dental Study Club, Spear Education Faculty Study Club, and the Schuster Center for Professional Development and Performance Coach.*

*Dr. Isaacs earned Diplomate status from the American Board of Dental Sleep Medicine. She has extensive training in cosmetic and restorative dentistry, including restoring dental implants and oral appliance therapy for sleep apnea. Her training includes ongoing study at Spear Education and the Schuster Center.*

*Dr. Isaacs is an Affiliated Clinical Assistant Professor in the Department of Operative Dentistry at the University of Florida and is a Spear Education Visiting Faculty Mentor in Scottsdale, Arizona.*

*Dr. Isaacs has been married to her soulmate, Tony, for 37 years, and has two daughters, Olivia and Michaela. Her leisure activities include spending time with her family, various church activities, Eucharistic Minister to the Sick, studio cycling, kayaking, boating, photography, yoga, and just about anything outside.*

*http://www.Drmaryisaacs.com*

# Chapter Nineteen
# Dr. Mike Robichaux
## Slidell, Louisiana

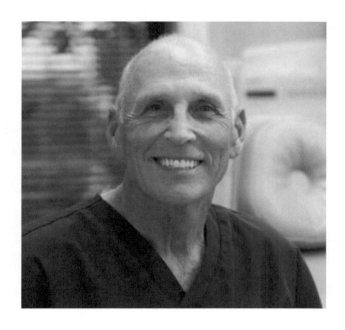

*The three-day case presentation seminar really opened my eyes to a better way to practice dentistry and to live my life. The first day Dr. Schuster asked us, "Why does your practice exist?" I got a little angry and huffy because I had a lot of debt, a home mortgage, a family to support, and lots of responsibility. At that time, I felt the purpose of my practice was to support my lifestyle.*

*Mike worked with the dentists in the class to help us understand that to be happy, the purpose of our practice had to be for the well-being of those we served. It was a game changer...*

## Early Practice, Clinical Continuing Education, and a Production Model

I graduated in the first class from Louisiana State University School of Dentistry in New Orleans. After graduation, I felt consciously incompetent. I didn't know enough to take good care of people, so I pursued lots of continuing education in clinical dentistry, 200-400 hours a year. My wife used to ask me, "Why are you so unhappy and restless?" I told her I wasn't unhappy but that I realized I didn't know enough. I spent two years in the Navy, and I traveled to study with several top dental educators like Pete Dawson, Alvin Fillastre, Harold Wirth, LD Pankey, and the Society for Occlusal Studies.

In the early 1980s, I joined Quest, a practice management program. I developed a large production-based practice with twelve employees. We found that many patients didn't like that style of practice and longed for a slower-paced practice which they had grown to love. I had developed what I thought I wanted, but when I got there, it wasn't for us.

One day my closest mentor, Dr. Harold Wirth asked me how things were going. I told him great, that we were growing in production and new patient flow, and that we were building a new building. Then he said, "Mike, are you getting any gifts? Are you

252

getting any thank you notes with the payment checks? Are you getting hugs?"

I answered, "No."

"Well, then you're not doing very well Mike."

It is easy when growing a new practice to begin seeing patients as sources for fulfilling our "requirements," i.e., meeting overhead, paying off debts, and funding our lifestyles. Little did I realize at the time how devastating that was in my quest to build a safe place for patients to receive dental care.

I believe a mentor chooses the mentee. Harold saw that I was serious, and he chose me. He helped me clarify my values and develop a vision for my practice. He helped me develop confidence that I could practice in a patient-centered way. He told me a dentist's job is to help people want what they need. I felt that was a higher road. We continued to see a significant number of patients leave the practice following the Review of Findings visit.

## Getting Organized with a Patient-Centered, Less-is-More Model

Dr. Wirth died in 1987, and a year later I heard Dr. Mike Schuster lecture at the first F. Harold Wirth Memorial Lecture at the

New Orleans Dental Conference. I had never heard a dentist speak like he did. I felt like he was talking directly to me. I joined the Schuster Center sometime later as a student. I learned quickly how to get control of time and money, and how to use systems to run the practice.

However, it was the three-day case presentation seminar that really opened my eyes to a better way to practice dentistry and to live my life. The first day Dr. Schuster asked us, and again I felt like he was speaking directly to me, "Why does your practice exist?" I got a little angry and huffy because I had a lot of debt, a home mortgage, a family to support, and lots of responsibility. At that time, I thought the purpose of my practice was to support my lifestyle.

Over the year in the Management course, Mike worked with the dentists in the class to help us understand that to be happy the purpose of our practice had to be for the well-being of those we served. It was a game-changer. I began to see things differently. My practice grew in maturity. By that I mean the size of the practice shrunk, and staff size decreased from normal attrition. However, profitability and the quality of patient care went up. I must have attended the Case Presentation Seminar eight times, and I served as a mentor for the class for many years.

# Refinement with Holistic, Health-Centered Care

In the mid-1990s, I discovered I had some kidney problems. My father had similar issues. I met Sam Queen, a biochemist, researcher, clinical nutritionist, and teacher. Thanks to Sam my kidneys are normal today. Working to get myself healthy and studying with Sam for twenty years gave me a different perspective on health and the nature of the disease. I gained an appreciation for how the mouth is related to our general health. That began another part of my professional journey.

Prevention and optimal health became a big part of the practice. We began a marketing program to attract patients who felt as we did, i.e., that the health of the mouth and our overall health are intimately related. That idea was key to the tremendous success that followed. It starts with the new patient interview--finding out what the patient wants, and how they want their mouth to be when they are eighty years old. Once they get clear on what they want then it's easy to show them disease in their mouth.

I tell new patients, "You're in a health-centered practice so we believe that each of us is responsible for our own health, you for you, me for me. So, if the hygienist tells you that your gums bleed, you need to pick up the mirror and ask her 'what do I need to do to stop this?' That's the way our practice works. We always assume that you want to be well."

We don't lecture or preach because it doesn't work. We don't tell people how to brush if they don't ask. Our mantra is "We help people move toward wellness." I share that with them before we go into the exam room, making sure they understand what we are all about. After the exam, I'll pick up a toothbrush and ask--I always ask for permission first, "Is it ok for me to show you what we think is the best way to take care of your mouth?" If patients don't want to move toward wellness, they don't do well in our office.

Many of the people coming to our office have health issues and were disappointed in their medical care because they weren't being told the cause of their problems. In their quest to learn more about their illness, they kept reading how they had to make sure their mouths were healthy. They find that if they don't get their mouth healthy, they can't get medically healthy either. These people want complete, systematic care, not patchwork repair and just treating symptoms. They want their mouth to be healthy and not deteriorate with age.

I always share with patients the "Secret" to stopping the deterioration of their mouths is to first, have no inflammation or infections in gums and bone around the teeth. Second, is to have no opening in any tooth that allows bacteria to enter the teeth. Third, to provide an inability of teeth to touch during sleep (accomplished with a nighttime bite appliance.)

Excellent daily dental care can produce a mouth that has no disease or pain, excluding of course pain caused by a dysfunctional chewing system. It is about first putting the fires out. As Dr. Schuster said many times, you don't call a carpenter until you have put the fires out. It's a wonderful gift to give to our patients who may only be able to afford care in phases and/or who are suffering from major medical conditions. Of course, we should seek to learn as much as possible about the entire orthognathic system and to develop skills that allow us to take a mouth apart and put it back together into a condition that would create stability for a very long time.

In 2005 Hurricane Katrina hit Louisiana. I was injured in an accident from a falling tree. I couldn't practice for a year during my recovery, but I never missed a payroll thanks to disability insurance and the concept of solvency (business savings) account established during my Schuster training. The following year I had another health issue that was life threatening. Those two episodes made me realize how precious each day was to me. As I sat on the edge of my bed preparing to go back to work after this second episode and feeling some anxiety about what the future had in store for me, I had a life-changing moment.

## Professional Service

I made the decision that I would become an advocate for my patients. I decided I wouldn't try to get them to do what I thought they needed to do for their mouths. Instead, it made sense to me to begin, as L.D. Pankey used to say, to know my patients! I'd find out what it is that they wanted for their mouth. What were their goals and values relative to their dental health? I'd ask them to gaze into the future and imagine what they wanted their mouths to be like when they were in their later years. It was magical. Many had trouble answering that question so often I'd ask them things like, "First, would it be important to keep your teeth?" Then, "Would you like to be free of infections, disease, and pain?" and "Would you like to eat whatever you wanted and be able to smile freely?" Of course, everyone answered yes to all these questions.

Then came the comprehensive exam where they learned about their mouths at the same time we did. It too was magical. Routinely they would ask the dental assistant when I left the room why no one had ever told them what they just heard. I always made a point before they left, to assure them that they were going to be fine and not to worry and that at the Review of Findings (ROFs) visit, it would all make sense.

The ROFs went from a highly structured visit to two individuals who respected each other having a cup of coffee and discussing something very important. I made a point to keep things from getting too complicated and confusing the patient. Most of the patients that left me early on no doubt were confused and wondered if they really needed all that we discussed. One thing, for sure, really helped. I became a master of photography, which proved invaluable in allowing the patients to comprehend exactly what was happening to their mouths. Along with this, we created a library of before and after photos of similar cases that they could use to see what their result would resemble. At the end of the visit, I'd give them a summary of what we discussed, attempted to answer all their questions and all the options that were before them. One of which was to do nothing. Invariably they would choose the most appropriate treatment based on their personal life circumstances and the one I would have recommended to them…how ironic! The level of trust that was created was off the charts! It made our office a very safe place for our patients, and they truly appreciated this approach.

What we have evolved into over 20-25 years is a minimally invasive, aggressively conservative, patient-centered, holistically inclined, general practice of dentistry. We were committed to excellence and patient care at a high level. We had about 1,100 patients and we would see one patient at a time. It's small and we have time for fun. The joy of going to work on Monday was still there when we retired. I know many people believe you can't have a small practice, but we did, and dentistry has provided us with a very comfortable lifestyle.

We had four employees plus my wife worked part-time. When we retired, all the members of my staff had been with me for 30 or more years with one over 40 years. If we were to write down the five most important things in our lives, they would probably be the same for all of us. We have philosophical congruence.

I haven't hired a new employee in many years. I believe the interview process is a poor predictor in determining if the applicant will be a good fit. Also, I don't believe previous experience is that important. We were looking at the heart and soul of the person. They didn't have to be in perfect fitness and health, but they did have to be health and fitness oriented. Being on that journey was enough. It's interesting to look back on the development of healthy habits over the last 30 years for the entire team, including myself. There is a psychological testing instrument to assess an applicant's emotional intelligence and values that can give tremendous insights into whether an applicant will succeed within an office.

I worked hard to treat my staff with dignity and respect. I treated them the way I wanted them to treat our patients, and that's what they did. The relationship with one's staff is one of the most important elements of a patient-centered practice. They have told me they don't work for me; they work for our patients. I didn't micromanage, and they appreciated the autonomy they had. I didn't do year-end reviews. Rather, if something happens, we will talk about it the first chance we get. The staff appreciated the openness and transparency we had amongst each other. Patients sensed it and it just permeated the whole office. We had half a day and sometimes all-day staff meetings to start every year. I asked them to tell me if they saw me acting for my own benefit at their expense or the expense of our patients. They always answered "No" for all those years, so I quit asking them.

Dentists mistakenly believe that advanced technical training and clinical courses will lead patients to accept treatment recommendations. That's not the case at all. I understand the problem from my own experience, and because I served as a director of the group that led the CE Department at LSUSD for many years. Success in a dental practice requires a three-pronged approach that happened simultaneously throughout my career:

1. Personal Growth: Even growing up in a normal family, it's common to develop limiting beliefs about ourselves. Early on I listened to Dr. Robert Schuller (he built the Crystal Cathedral in California), Norman Vincent Peale, and others speaking about personal growth. I read books by James

Allen…As a Man Thinketh, M. Scott Peck…The Road Less Traveled, and many more. All that studying, looking back, allowed me to become more genuine which greatly enhanced the trust we have in our patients.

2. Clinical Skills: I was blessed to have the awareness that I didn't know enough and that my clinical skills were deficient if I was going to practice dentistry at a high level. Having a wife who was diagnosed with deteriorating condyles in 1973, the year after I graduated provided the real impetus to learn more. Having patients with debilitating dental issues is one thing but when one works and lives with them…now that is another story. From Pete Dawson to Alvin Fillastre to Bernie Williams, to Bill Farrar…they were all giants. I loved to go to meetings, learn new things, and at the same time getting to hang out with some wonderful clinicians who were sitting right next to me. I often learned as much visiting with guys and gals who freely shared what they were doing as I did in the lectures. Getting CE at home via video can be helpful but much is lost by not being around exciting people.

3. People Skills: The ability to be with people, and to help them make good decisions came from my own transformation. It comes from connecting to who we are, why we're here, and what we are trying to do with our lives. What do we want people to say at our funeral? What do we want our children

to hear when they are in the grocery store and a former patient comes up to them? What is our life about? Is it about accumulating things? If we come from a place of fear, there will never be enough. We'll try to go faster, and we'll want more things and bigger things. I believe if we come from a place of love, life is different and much better. If we see abundance, then there will always be enough. We can't help another without helping ourselves. Less is really more. We go slower so that we can go faster.

It bothers me that we're losing the belief that we can make a fine living dedicating ourselves to helping people. We can have a healthy, wonderful life. We don't have to use people, manipulate them, or sell things and push people to do things so that we can get more toys. A worldview based on service is very important and it comes from within and from the clarification of our value system.

As we were winding down a fifty-plus-year career in dentistry, utilizing the principles outlined above, we inadvertently got busier. It was what we were seeking back in 1974 when we started. How sad it took so long to learn these things. It was a great ride. We touched many souls. We even fixed a lot of mouths.

*Dr. Mike Robichaux began practicing dentistry in Slidell, LA in 1974. Over the subsequent 40+ years, Dr. Robichaux would amass over 4,000 hours of continuing dental education. He would also befriend and work closely with accomplished health professionals who sought to achieve health on the molecular level. It was through Dr. Robichaux's deep understanding of the connection between oral health and overall health that he created a truly unique approach to dentistry, and it is this approach that serves as the backbone of his practice's philosophy.*

# Chapter Twenty
# Dr. Jack King
## Statesville, North Carolina

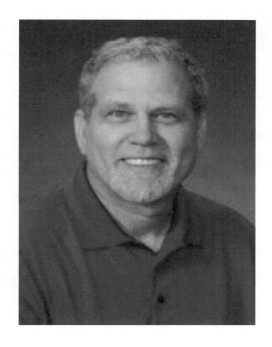

*The best thing that happened was a surprise! Everything I did with the Schuster Center was out of my comfort zone. But I discovered that if I got out of my comfort zone, positive things could result from that!*

*I started to realize that the way I and my team interacted with patients influenced the choices they made, especially in a way that would benefit them long term.*

*The Schuster Center is a pathway to building a life that you want to have.*

265

# Startup Practice, Getting Busy and Frustrated

I have wanted to be a dentist since I was fourteen years old. I knew I wanted to be in health care, and help people, and I liked working with my hands. I worked at a golf course in high school, and I met several dentists. My own dentist was a great golfer. They were very nice to me, and they seemed more friendly than the physicians at the golf course.

My father influenced me as well. He was an accountant in a small manufacturing company. He had multiple horrible bosses who made his work life miserable. He encouraged my sister and me to attend graduate school and find a career where we would have control over our lives. I wanted to be my own boss so I could be in charge of my life. I figured dentistry would provide a good life for my family appropriate for me given my education, intelligence, and motivation. It would give me a chance to use my people skills, work with my hands, and build a quality life.

I graduated from the University of North Carolina Chapel Hill Dental School in 1983, and I started a practice from scratch in the small town of Statesville where I grew up. My banker helped me find a dental office space with two operatories. Later, I bought a bigger office next door, but I was in the same parking lot for thirty-two years.

I didn't know much about running a business or practicing dentistry for that matter. I listened to popular practice management speakers at the time, Linda Miles, Burt Press, and Dwayne Smith, who promoted the "Million Dollar Practice." They all advocated increasing production and busyness, which I didn't have. I figured I should get busy, and getting busy would mean I was successful.

Two and a half years later I was disturbed, distraught, and frustrated. I had gotten busy doing what the experts suggested. I was running back and forth between two operatories, and I was doing all the hygiene myself. I didn't hire a hygienist until two years later. I was doing a lot of single tooth, repair dentistry—taking a tooth out here, doing a filling or a crown there, and a partial denture there. I was just bouncing around with very little organization in my life.

Now that I've been on a lifelong curve of trying to figure out who I am and what's important, I've come to understand that I'm not good at chaos. I function better, and I'm happier with a sense of order. Back then I had none of that.

## Clinical Training at the Pankey Institute

I shared my frustration with my childhood dentist, who was a Pankey-trained dentist. He said, "Jack, you need to go to the Pankey Institute." I started taking courses at the Pankey Institute in 1986. I thought here's a philosophy that is more like what I should be doing. I should treat the whole patient, and I should slow down and start to think about my practice differently.

I went back home and tried to implement Pankey-style dental care without leadership and communication skills. I only had the clinical skills I had learned. For example, patients' jaws should be in a certain position. If you accomplish that then you are a good dentist. If you neglect correct jaw positioning, then you are a terrible dentist and you should turn in your license and go pump gas somewhere. That was the way I understood it, and I don't think I was the only one to get that message.

A year later Dr. Mike Schuster's flyer came across my desk. I thought, here's a dentist who taught at the Pankey Institute so he should understand the philosophy of care and slowing down the practice. My wife, Carol, went with me to Charlotte to attend Mike's course. The seminar was partly about personal and business financial organization, and partly about practice management. I remember thinking, this is the guy for me. He taught a model of practice that matched up with what I needed to know about running my practice with the higher level of dental care that I aspired to deliver. It would help me get a sense of order and control in the practice day in and day out. I knew if I had that I would be better off.

Mike came to North Carolina again about six months later to speak to the Academy of General Dentistry. At the break, I invited him to meet so we could talk about dentistry. He agreed and the next morning we went for a run together. I told him my dad (the accountant) had been helping me track the numbers in the practice as he advised in the previous class seven months prior. I said, "It's been really helpful, and I feel like I'm on the path now to being the best dentist I can be."

He asked me, "Would you be willing to stand up in front of the class at the next break and tell the group what you've learned?" I was nervous about that, but I agreed.

I watched for Mike whenever he was teaching on the East Coast. I attended another class about a year later, and I met an analyst from the Schuster Center, Blair Kolkowski. I learned Dr. Schuster had a one-year Management Program. Blair came out to my office and did a thorough assessment, called a Practice Health Evaluation. At the end of the assessment, I wrote a big check to enroll in the Management course.

## Getting Organized with the Schuster Center

I wanted to slow down and organize my practice around Pankey clinical care. I wanted to improve how I managed staff. We had no team meetings and no morning huddles.

First, we learned how money flowed in the practice, and then policies and systems for administration. Everything was discussed, then documented and written down.

Everything was hard for me because of where I was in my life at that time. I was anxious about change and speaking in front of groups. Traveling to Arizona with my team was difficult. Monthly coaching calls with the Schuster Center helped manage progress in incremental steps over the year.

The best thing that happened was a surprise! Everything I did with the Schuster Center was out of my comfort zone. But I discovered that if I got out of my comfort zone, positive things could result from that!

However, I took easily to tracking the numbers, i.e., the key performance indicators of the practice. That gave me a sense of control, knowing how the money was flowing in and out of the practice. During the first five years of practice, I barely understood what accounts receivables were. Also, tracking the numbers gave me a task to do with my dad and tap into his expertise.

The first treatment planning, case presentation session was a turning point for me. We went from a one-appointment new patient exam to two visits. In addition, for four years the first visit was an interview that was free of charge. The second visit was the clinical exam, and the third visit was the Review of Findings consultation. Later on, we combined the interview with the clinical exam, so the new patient process was just two appointments. This process helped me slow down, ask questions, listen better, and try to help people think about their future in a proactive manner.

That's when I really started to realize that the way I and my team interacted with patients influenced the choices they made, especially in a way that would benefit them long term. We dedicated our practice to helping people maintain their natural dentition in an optimum state of health, comfort, and function for life.

As we wrote down our vision, mission, and policies/systems we started having regular weekly meetings and morning huddles. The team went with me to the Schuster Center for seminars and they all supported the new practice vision and structure. It was exciting. In fact, they all stayed with the practice for twenty-plus years after we started the program.

I became a believer in how important it is to help people get healthy. I read Bob Barkley's book, *Successful Preventive Dental Practices,* listened to his tapes, and implemented the Dental Fitness Program in hygiene and the new patient process. I thought deeply about helping patients accept responsibility for their health, and how to protect teeth from fracture or breakdown over their life. My belief in the philosophy of health and protecting teeth led to personal action. I had my entire mouth restored by Dr. Sam Davis, an associate faculty at the Pankey Institute, and I paid the full fee for it.

My overhead decreased steadily over the subsequent years and then stabilized at 52% for the duration. So, profitability was excellent. Initially, that was important for me. But quickly, maybe in two to three years, it just became less important. I had become friends with Blair, the analyst who did my PHE, and we talked frequently. I referred many of my dental colleagues to Blair for a PHE.

At his wedding reception, Blair and I were chatting, and I told him, "You know Blair, I don't have much money right now, but I have a plan, and I have developed the discipline to implement the plan, so I'm just going to go ahead and start acting like I already have that money that I anticipate having when I'm fifty-six years old."

Things worked out closely to that plan. I wanted my net worth to be four million dollars when I retired. I don't know where that number came from, it just seemed reasonable. So, I put the plan in place, and I just quit being anxious about money.

I teach a financial literacy class here at UNC Dental School. I tell the dental students, "The primary goal is for you to have a healthy relationship with money, and that has nothing to do with how much money you have. It has to do with the way you think about money and the psychology of money that you choose to adopt. If you don't have a realistic psychology about what money is, what it can and can't do, and how you can best interact with it, you'll never get over being anxious about money. That's true no matter how much money you have."

## Practice Refinement with the CEO Program

As we became more organized and effective, I added staff. I continued with coaching from the Schuster Center for two years after the Management Program. It was called the CEO program. The practice grew, and profit was steady and excellent. But then we got too busy again.

I had never been in a network with insurance companies, but if patients had dental insurance, we accepted the assignment of benefits and waited for insurance to pay before we collected the patient portion. In 1991 I told the team, "All right you all, we're going to wean ourselves off the dental insurance business. We'll assign insurance benefits directly to the patient, and we won't accept any checks from insurance companies. If they send us a check, we'll send it back to the insurance company."

Obviously, we had to build value with patients to take responsibility for their health and well-being. Part of that was helping them understand their financial obligation and be willing to commit to that, knowing that some of that money would come back to them from the insurance company.

At that time, I had a second full-time hygienist who decided not to return to work after her maternity leave. That was fine with me as I was tired of checking two rooms of hygiene patients anyway. It was the right mix of how things happen sometimes. We had about 2,500 active patients, and we went through a patient qualification process. Every month my team and I went through one-twelfth of the charts and reviewed our patients. We didn't always agree on how each patient qualified as the right fit for our practice.

"C" patients were uncooperative patients who didn't pay their bills, failed their appointments, and didn't follow through with their treatment plans. They accounted for about four hundred patients and most of the disruptive emergencies. I sent them a letter explaining we no longer had the services of a second hygienist for their preventive therapy. I explained we would be happy to see them for emergencies for one month, and we would be happy to send their records to the dentist of their choice for no charge.

"B" patients were the middle eight hundred patients of the practice, cooperative patients who were growable, but didn't take full responsibility for their oral health. I sent a different letter to them explaining the reduced hygiene capacity and that we couldn't honor their current appointment. However, if they would be flexible and give us some time, we would get them into the schedule. If they were at all uncomfortable with that, we would forward their records to the dentist of their choice at no charge.

"A" patients were the most cooperative and loyal patients in the practice. They accounted for 20-40% of the patient population. They referred other patients, paid their bills on time, kept their appointments, and followed through with their treatment plans. We sent them a letter telling them how wonderful they were and how much we enjoyed working with them. I explained they might hear about changes we made in the practice, but they would not be affected by those changes at all, and we hoped they would stay with us as long as the practice exists.

Beyond getting organized, slowing down, and getting control of money, the intangible benefits of the Management were even greater. I enjoyed seeing my team work better and feel better about being at work every day.

The Schuster Center gave me control over my work environment, and it helped me build a financial plan. I knew economic freedom was the result if I lived long enough to execute the plan. It gave me the freedom to travel on the weekends, to prepare for teaching Sunday school, to volunteer at the local women's shelter, and to be with my family. In many ways, I've had blessings that make me want to share some of what I've learned.

## Mentoring and Coaching at the Schuster Center

After the CEO program, I stayed connected to the Schuster Center as a mentor, and I referred many dentists there. Mike got tired of flying all over the country two weekends a month and he engaged me and two other mentors, Don Trunkey, and Cary LaCouture, to start doing some of the one-day seminars. I stuck with it the longest, about twenty years off and on. I had been helped in such a positive way that I wanted to share that with my friends and the public at large. I made that choice consciously and it was a big step in my personal growth and development to lecture a group of my peers for 7-8 hours about dentistry and what I'd learned. It was very much a step beyond anywhere I ever dreamed I would be, but the Schuster Center had been very valuable for me and my friends. I was extremely nervous about giving the first seminar. I figured it would be a growth experience for me, and I believed it was valuable material for other dentists. Even if they didn't enroll in the Schuster

Center Management Program it would be valuable for them to go back home and track the numbers as I'd done.

Eventually, Mike and I spent time discussing if I would be the next one to manage the Schuster Center when he slowed down, but that didn't work out. But I stayed connected for a time after that and Mike had me doing coaching calls with eight to nine dentists a month.

## Leaving Active Practice to Teach

About ten years ago I suddenly developed an autoimmune disease, Polymyalgia Rheumatica, after a day of hard manual labor in the sun. It froze mobility in my shoulders, hips, and neck, and practicing dentistry was painful. I did four months of medical tests and took steroids and strong medication for two years. But it never resolved, and I realized I couldn't work in the practice anymore. I was fifty-six years old.

I met with my financial advisor. I asked him, "It's not what I planned, but what would happen if I retired now?" He said, "You know how to manage your life and your spending so if that's what you need to do, we'll help you make it work."

I put my practice up for sale and sold it to a young dentist who wanted the type of practice I had. I knew I couldn't do dentistry, but I also knew I wasn't done working. I was already volunteering to teach part-time in the clinic at the dental school. That was easy for me.

I worked with Paragon Dental Transition Company for a year and a half. They told me, "You know more about how dental practices work than anyone at the company. We need a VP here on the East Coast." But none of the dentists I consulted wanted to sell their practice. I was shocked at how little they knew about their practices. They didn't know what their revenue was, what their overhead was, and they didn't even know if they had a 401K. They were oblivious. I knew I couldn't work in that environment.

Gradually, over two years at the dental school, I went from part-time to full-time in 2017. I never expected to be a full-time professor. My main role is supervision in the clinic, and not long ago I took over the practice management course.

Teaching the students and helping them think about their future in a different way, is the greatest life experience that I've had. For the last seven to eight years, I've been on a mission, and I'll execute that mission for as long as my health and well-being allow. Many students are going to work in corporate practices because that's where the jobs are. They know that I'm from the private practice, fee-for-service world and that I never engaged with an insurance company. We have lots of talks about being in or out of network. I encourage them to fully seek freedom and autonomy.

I tell them from day one "Here's the number one thing. You must find a place to work that gives you the opportunity to do the very best dentistry that you're capable of doing. A lot of places you go are not going to care about how good of a job you do. They're going to be interested in the revenue that you can generate for their private equity investment firm. Therefore, if they don't give you the time and freedom to treat your patients as you know is best, then you must move on. Your first job won't be your last job."

I've learned to see myself for who I am and to be more forgiving to myself and others for being imperfect. I've been strongly influenced by my religious upbringing and the way I saw my parents behave in the community. I thought we were lucky. We were never wealthy, but we had food on the table and a roof over our heads. I always felt like, despite all the problems in my life, that I had a special blessing. It doesn't obligate me, but it makes me want to give back and I can't say why.

I like to be in control of things, but I've given up trying to control everything. I put my best effort into the situation, and then I let the outcome be what it is. The Schuster Center is a pathway to building a life that you want to have. Its long hard work that you must do, but it can be a pathway out of the forest into the light. For me it absolutely was.

*Dr. Jack King owned his dental practice in Statesville, NC from 1983 to 2015. Currently, he is an Associate Professor at the University Of North Carolina Chapel Hill School of Dentistry, where he's been faculty for eight years.*

# Chapter Twenty-One
# Dr. Jim Sandlin
## Duluth, Georgia

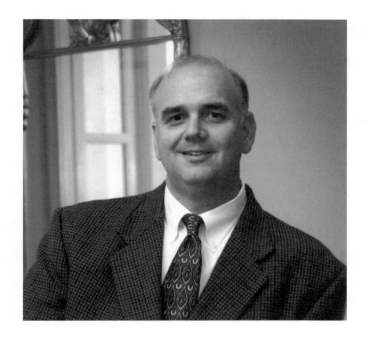

*I would tell young dentists they need to clear out the noise in their lives so they can hear themselves think. Get control of their time and their finances to make room for what they could become. They need to grow personally and develop a clear picture of who they are. They need to focus on their vision, what they want, and why they want it.*

## Starting From Scratch

I've wanted to be a dentist since I was six years old. Dentistry seemed like a great career in which I could help people, be my own boss, and create something with my hands. My family went to a wonderful dentist while I was growing up. His was a small family office and my goal was to have a similar relationship-based practice when I started. I wanted my patients to feel safe, not experience pain, and receive quality care.

In 1983 I graduated from Emory University Dental School and was hired as an associate in a family practice. But I was eager to have my own office. In late 1984, I decided to start from scratch in Duluth, GA, a fast-growing suburb of Atlanta. I paid cash for everything I could and only borrowed for good, but very basic equipment. My wife was the family provider for the first year. She was a pediatric ICU nurse.

## Frustration with a Production Model and Expert Consultants

The practice grew quickly, and we broke even after four months. After one year, I had one part-time and three full-time employees. After two years, we were even busier, but it became obvious that I didn't know how to manage a business. It was chaos.

We had few office systems. We could only react to problems as they came up. I attended lectures at state dental meetings to hear speakers like Jim Pride and Linda Miles, hoping to learn how to run a successful practice. During those first years, I tried every dental and non-dental consulting firm I could afford, hoping a better organization would solve my stress and frustration. They all told me the same thing—produce more, get busier, and do more marketing.

Production went up, but that brought even more problems. My stress increased. I was miserable. Patient communications focused on memorized scripts meant to generate more production. Some local dentist friends were going to the Pankey Institute or Dawson for advanced training to "fix" their practices. They spent lots of time and money, but I saw little change in their practices or their lives. It didn't seem like a good investment for me.

I then completed a three-year business course in leadership and management. We developed tools for improved hiring and office communication. After all that, I still didn't see real improvement in my practice. Staff problems only grew worse. I hired people for their personality type and great skills, but it was hit-and-miss. I'd hire a good staff member but then I'd hire someone who would run off the good one. It was churn and burn and replace another staff member every six months.

By my fifteenth year in practice, I had a staff of ten and a custom-built 3,000-square-foot office. From the outside things looked great. My patient base was growing, and production numbers were decent. Inside I hated going to work. I had no financial stability and I found no happiness in my practice.

One morning, I drove to the office in my beat-up truck and noticed all the other cars in staff parking were brand new. It was like everyone else was getting ahead at my expense, while I was falling behind. At that moment, I was ready to pull the plug and walk away, just to get out. I thought to myself, "I'm going to rent bikes on the beach. It's got to be more fun than this!"

## Management Program at the Schuster Center

Fortunately, Dr. Jeff Foltz, a friend from my church group, convinced me to wait six months before selling out and try working with the Schuster Center for Professional Development. They performed a Practice Health Evaluation, and an analyst showed me how the SC could help. His plan looked great, but I had no savings or cash flow to pay the tuition he proposed. Plus, my wife doubted another "consultant" was going to be any different from all the others we had tried. I almost walked away.

Nevertheless, I took a leap of faith and enrolled in the Management Course, hoping I could find a way to afford it. I wanted to exhaust all possibilities before giving up and leaving dentistry. Right away the SC helped me control accounts receivable. Four months into the program I saw that my bills were paid and there was money left over. I also paid off the SC tuition in those four months! I thought, "Wow, this really works!"

During Management I gained clarity and personal commitment to my vision. This led to hiring better people and developing a staff closely aligned with where I wanted to go. I continued with classes at the Schuster Center after the Management course, and I attended several three-day alumni conferences. I worked on my leadership skills, the new patient process, and treatment consultations. It took me three years to get truly organized and become effective with a Review of Findings. In addition, I had to keep upgrading my office systems to keep pace with the higher level of treatment my patients were asking for. My patients had begun to trust me.

## Continued Improvement with a Performance Coach and a Niche Practice

Five years after Management I enrolled in Performance Coach (PC). I wanted more of the powerful coaching, increased profitability, and improved team dynamics I'd experienced in the Management Course. We spent time in reflection, goal setting, studying the nature of health, and refining our practices. I got to know myself more clearly and discovered what was holding me back. Performance Coach helped me evaluate my progress and determine the next best step to develop myself and my practice. Near the end of PC, Dr. Schuster advised me I was now ready for advanced training in restorative dentistry and occlusion. Since Pankey and Dawson didn't click for me, Dr. Schuster recommended that I attend OBI.

My story demonstrates that you can have a lot of management tools, but if you don't understand why, how, and when to use them, it really doesn't matter. When I came to the SC I had tools, but I understood them at a basic level, and I didn't know how to release their power.

Over the last ten years, the practice has rocked. I've ramped up my success treating TMD patients and have built administrative and clinical systems to support this niche. The Schuster Center taught me the principles, strategies, and methods to bring my practice into alignment with a clear vision. I love it. I'm a general dentist who has developed a practice that gets referrals from the medical community as well as from other dentists.

I guess it goes back to why I chose dentistry and my desire to create good experiences for patients. I'm not looking to just

"Drill, fill, and bill". Where my strengths lie, my sweet spot, and what brings me energy, is sitting with patients who have gone from doctor to doctor and never found answers. I help them discover their current condition and together we discover what's causing their problem. Then, through the new patient process, we together establish their health goals and develop a treatment plan to support their unique needs. The SC gave me the freedom to grow into the professional I've wanted to become.

## Financial Independence and Giving Back to Dentistry

A few years after completing the Management course, Paula and I were financially independent. All our debts were paid, and we had cash to invest in the future. During COVID-19, I realized we had everything in place for retirement. I could keep practicing if I wanted, but I didn't have to. I chose to sell my office in 2022 and I currently work part-time (just for fun) consulting TMJ patients in other doctors' practices.

Paula and I are enjoying life. We've taken bicycle trips all over the world. Last year we cycled across the western US from Seattle to Yellowstone Park. This year we're riding through Tuscany. Next Spring, we plan to cycle across Japan and Korea to see the cherry blossoms.

I would tell young dentists they need to clear out the noise in their lives so they can hear themselves think. Get control of their time and their finances to make room for what they could become. They need to grow personally and develop a clear picture of who they are. They need to focus on their vision, what they want, and why they want it.

The Cheshire Cat was right, "If you don't know where you're going, any road will take you there".

*Dr. Jim Sandlin and his wife Paula divide their time between Duluth and Tybee Island, GA. They have four adult children and one super adorable granddaughter.*

*Here's a letter Dr. Sandlin recently sent to Dr. Schuster:*

*Mike,*

*I've wanted to write you for several months. Last January, I sold part of my practice and limited my care to OBI-type rehab cases. Then, in mid-May, I took time off completely to reflect and decide what I wanted to "be" in this second half of life. (Maybe "last quarter" is more accurate.)*

*Paula and I traveled to Portugal in May/June and bicycled the Portuguese Camino de Santiago. When we returned home, we repacked our bags and cycled from Seattle to Yellowstone over another 6 weeks. It was a great experience and gave me a lot of time to reflect on my 40 years in dentistry. During the many hours of riding/walking up the Cascades, you and the Center kept coming to mind.*

*Thank you for helping me grow up. I was a mess when I first arrived in Phoenix. Management year helped me clear the fog I had created with bad decisions. It took several years afterward to start cleaning myself up, but in retrospect, I had to grow into a person who could handle the next steps.*

*I know that I was the only one in the initial Performance Coach who had not completed Mastery. Thank you for allowing me to participate. PC gave me a group within which I could develop. Friends like John Herrin and Cree Hamilton helped me do the inside work I needed. Also, the hours we spent with Jim Hollis helped me understand myself better and gave me the tools to create a life I didn't know I could have.*

*Management helped create space in my life and PC helped me fill that space with what I was really supposed to become.*

*Thank you for challenging me to complete OBI. By the 1990s the Pankey and Dawson experiences weren't attracting me like they did when I first graduated. I don't know why, but while my friends were traveling to Florida and nothing really changed in their lives,*

*I wanted to work on my communication and leadership skills. That's how I landed at the Center. OBI came into my life at the right time. It gave me what I was looking for when I felt I could use it.*

*Please know that your encouragement has allowed me to influence, in a small way, the care patients are provided in a lot of places. People in the southeast US, as well as Vietnam, are seeing their patients differently because of my OBI experience. Thank you for pointing me in that direction.*

*I'm now sorting things out about returning to limited practice versus putting everything on the shelf and turning to the relationships in my life outside of dentistry. I still haven't made up my mind. Thanks to the work I did at the Center, Paula and I have the financial means to create whatever life we choose. This is the freedom I was searching to find. Thank you.*

*You, your family, and everyone at the Center offered me hope when I didn't have much left. It wasn't always comfortable, but the work I needed to do was always put in front of me. For that, I'm eternally grateful.*

*Godspeed,*

*Jim*

# Chapter Twenty-Two
# Dr. Ivette Rodriguez
## Humacao, Puerto Rico

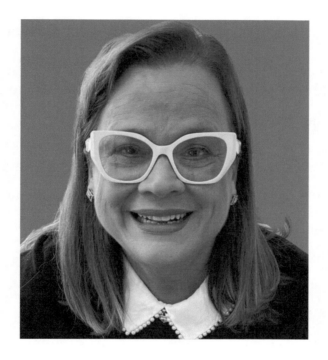

*My priority is to establish a relationship with the child and his or her parents. I embrace the child and often we cry together. I educate the parents and we must agree on prevention, or I won't accept them into the practice. That's the most important thing.*

## I Did What My Mother Said

As a little girl, I would often accompany my mother to her work. She taught microbiology at the medical school. I used to play with little white mice in the laboratory. I wanted to be like my mother. I told her I wanted to get a PhD and do research. She said it would be wiser to study dentistry and get my doctorate degree first. Then I could study whatever I wanted. I did what she told me, and I went to dental school.

I finished with no school debt because I had a scholarship, and my mom was teaching at the medical school. I graduated Magna cum Laude. I got married right after graduation. My husband is the best and dearest friend I ever had in my life. He is brilliant, benevolent, and unique. He's the wind behind my wings, and he supports me in whatever I want to do. Now, we've been married for forty-six years. We have four children who are in their forties now. My husband is an OB/GYN, so I had all my children for free.

## Poor Organization and Too Many Patients

I started my pediatric dental practice from scratch with four chairs and worked two days a week. My practice is in Humacao, Puerto Rico, a city of about 60,000 people. It's close to Palmas Del Mar, a resort community with 200,000 people in the surrounding area. I was pregnant when I first opened the practice, and I had all four children quickly in the next six years.

As the practice grew, I gradually added workdays until I was working full-time in a few years. I got too busy, and it was stressful to care for all the new patients coming to my office. People come to me from all over the island because no other dentists do what I do. I wanted to enjoy work more. I don't pay much attention to income, but I had to deal with the changing structure of medical care here. Puerto Rico is transitioning from private care to a Medicaid model. I wanted to decrease stress and get better organized. Further, I needed to figure out how I could serve patients in the Medicaid model and remain profitable. It's in my nature to be visionary and think about the future.

## Schuster Center Management Program

I heard about Dr. Schuster from another pediatric dentist in Orlando, FL. He recommended the Management Program to get my practice organized and profitable. He said I would not regret spending the time and money for the tuition and travel from Puerto Rico to Arizona. It was expensive to close the office and fly my staff to Arizona four times during the year.

My employees from that time are not with me anymore. However, my current staff have all been trained with the same policies and systems we developed at the Schuster Center, and they support my vision and philosophy. We operate the practice like a McDonald's franchise. Clinical and administrative procedures are planned and part of a consistent system. We have a morning huddle every day, and we regularly have a training meeting out of the office at a nice hotel. My staff appreciate how we care for patients, and I can tell they are happy to work here.

We set SMART goals which are specific, measurable, actionable, realistic, and time bound. Also, we set up percentage budgeting for expenses, doctor salary, and saving ten percent for ROI (return on investment.) I stopped spending carelessly and told my husband, "My god, look how much I saved in one year!"

Dr. Schuster was on leave from teaching at the Schuster Center when I started the program because he was recovering from back surgery. I didn't meet him until the end of the year. I learned a lot from Roberto, who taught many of the classes. I pushed him for as much information as I could get.

Eventually, I invited Dr. Schuster to Puerto Rico to stay at my home and explain his philosophy of care to my dental colleagues. We became friends and we appreciate each other's dedication and service to the profession. He's available for help when I need to call him. When Hurricane Maria caused severe damage in Puerto Rico, Dr. Schuster was the first one to call me.

One day I challenged Dr. Schuster regarding the Schuster Model. I said to him, "Of course, you have this beautiful practice, and people fly from all over to see you. But I'm in Puerto Rico, and it's not the same as Scottsdale, Arizona."

He told me, "It was similar for me in Wisconsin. My practice was in a farming community and people didn't have much money. But they valued what I was doing for them. We need to understand and appreciate what patients want and what they need. We are responsible for communicating that to them." So, I've learned to do that and to help people want what they need. I received a government grant to cover orthodontic treatment for people who can't afford the treatment.

Twenty-six years ago, I had an idea that I still hope to make real. I've kept all the manuals I received from the Management Program. I speak Spanish so I can teach the Schuster Model and his philosophy of care to dentists in Puerto Rico and South America.

## Benefits from the Management Program

I learned that if I'm organized with the right strategy, I can accomplish my goals. That's where the Schuster Center helped me the most. Most of my patients are handicapped, and many are young preschoolers. I can't rush with these patients, and I only see two to four patients a day. I'm careful to schedule adequate time for the interview, exam, education for the parents, and treatment for the child. I can't be interrupted during long procedures in the hospital, or when I'm treating children with sedation in the office.

I do everything for patients in two appointments. The first appointment is a consultation, exam, radiographs, and an estimate for treatment. However, my priority is to establish a relationship with the child and his or her parents. I embrace the child and often we cry together. I educate the parents and we must agree on prevention, or I won't accept them into the practice. That's the most important thing. Poor people find the money for treatment when they understand I want the best for their health. People tell me I'm cheerful, warm, and compassionate. I've been blessed with good communication skills since I was young.

I conducted workshops and taught leadership classes for years. So, I use the same emotional intelligence tools to build relationships with patients and families. A relationship of trust is the glue that binds us together. I tell people, "You are not just teeth, and you are not coming here for a dental cleaning. You are a human being and thank you for bringing your child to me. I'm here for the long term, and I'll take care of your child until my last day."

My assistant gives the parents an office tour and shows them the lab where we sterilize instruments. We explain that bagged instruments have been sterilized to prevent cross-infection. We explain that they will know how to evaluate any dental office. Then they sit down with me, and we talk and laugh. I give them a test and it goes something like this.

I say, "Have you ever had any cavities?"

They answer, "Yes, doctor."

I say, "Well, when you were born did you have any cavities?"

They answer, "No, doctor."

I say, "OK, now you have one minute to tell me five ways that you got those cavities. What habits did you have as a child?"

They always answer, "Candy." Then they start looking up at the ceiling which means they are accessing their memory. Often, they'll say, "Ugh, I don't know. I guess I didn't use my toothbrush at night."

I tell them, "OK, you got a D," and we start laughing. They are embarrassed and that's what I want. I want them out of their comfort zone, and a bit hurt. If they are out of their comfort zone, then they can start learning.

Then I ask a serious question, "Who taught you the habits you had as a child? We know cavities come from bad habits."

They say, "Oh, my mom taught me."

I tell them, "Look at your mother's mouth. She has cavities too. That means that the same information she gave you, which she got from her mother, you are going to give to your children. But now you will have my information and you can stop the cavities."

Then I explain how sealants work, and I review their oral hygiene. One thing that I do, and it's a great, great tool is I buy gallons of disclosing solution. I ask them when they last brushed their teeth and they'll say, "I brushed them this morning." Then I disclose their mouth and their teeth are all pink. They don't realize how poorly they remove plaque.

One patient went to another dentist in a nearby town, but then she returned to my office. She said, "He doesn't clean my teeth like you do in your office, and he doesn't use the red dye like you use so that everything gets white."

I told her, "Good for you. You put horns on me and went to another dentist, but now you understand why I do things a certain way." Some patients want me to do what they want, but I can't do that. I might please them once, but it comes back to cause bigger problems later. Eventually, patients understand, and they accept my philosophy. I have a high rate of acceptance for my treatment recommendations.

I do the exam and explain that if we eliminate the cavities, do sealants, and straighten their teeth with orthodontics then they won't have any more problems or toothaches. After the exam, I determine if the child will need sedation for the appointment. They leave the first appointment with an estimate of the cost of treatment, and they bring the money on the second appointment. Then I do all their treatment in one visit. I have four assistants with me in the clinical area. We pamper the patients while they are in the dental chair. For example, we often paint their nails and give them a pedicure.

I don't do external marketing or advertising, but I've received some free publicity. One handicapped child has been with me for twenty-six years. Her parents bring her to my office from an hour and a half away. Her father spoke to a reporter about how I've helped his daughter and one day a television news crew showed up at my office to do a documentary about my practice. I had to work on my days off for three months to handle all the new patients. That happened over two years ago, and I still have people coming in who say they saw me on the TV.

## The Future

I'm seventy-two now and it's time for me to slow down and focus on giving back. I found a pediatric dentist in Orlando who speaks Spanish and wants to work in my office. She shares my philosophy, and she enrolled in leadership workshops to develop her communication skills and people skills.

Currently, I'm vice president at the College of Dentistry in Puerto Rico. I declared that I will be president in 2025. I have a vision to improve dental care for elderly patients who are confined to a bed or wheelchair. I started a research project in March visiting geriatric patients. What we found was disappointing. Out of 461 patients, 26 had oral cancer, and 76 had advanced oral disease needing complex treatment in a hospital operating room. All these people have Medicaid, but there is no facility to treat them, and no dentists are prepared to treat them.

So, I'm starting a training program to address the needs of this population. First, is proper oral hygiene education for caregivers, then training for dentists. I am collaborating with politicians and Doctor Terry Graham from New York, who is recognized for his work in geriatric dentistry. Also, we have drafted

300

a law regarding this issue that will be presented to the senate. Elderly people deserve a basic quality of life in the last years of life.

I want everyone to pay it forward and help the less fortunate. We must have faith and do the work. Conversations are only thoughts. We must take action to obtain the result we want. Don't forget success comes from service, satisfaction, and remuneration in that order. I must enjoy the present in order to live with service, satisfaction, and remuneration.

*Dr. Ivette Rodríguez Quesada*

*Dr. Rodriguez has a motto, "Going to the dentist is fun."*

*Dr. Rodriguez Quesada graduated Magna Cum Laude from the School of Dental Medicine of the University of Puerto Rico in 1978. Her passion is patients with special needs and adults.*

*Dr. Rodriguez was trained in emotional intelligence, and she participated in a transformation company, Workshops for a New Lifestyle, for 17 years. She dedicates much of her practice to sedation related to her psychological knowledge to offer all dental treatment in a single appointment.*

# Chapter Twenty-Three
# Dr. Charlie Dingman
## Gillette, Wyoming

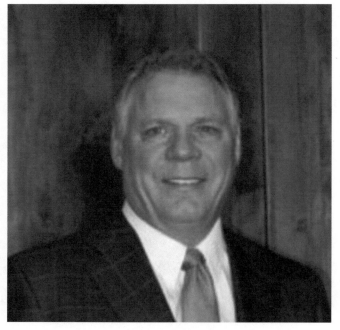

*I went from a small, slower-paced practice in Lincoln, NE to one that was very busy in Gillette, WY. We had too many patients, and the pace was hectic. Our goal was to slow it down so we could spend time with patients and give them the care and attention they deserved.*

*We cut our clinical hours, increased our production, decreased our overhead, and our net profit went up significantly. The staff size became more manageable, and the staff experienced more ownership and growth. We got control of time and money. Dr. Schuster's percentage budgeting made a dramatic difference!*

## Early Training and Challenges

I wanted to be a dentist since I was nine years old. My early dental experiences were very uncomfortable, and I didn't like going to the dentist. But one day I had an experience that changed my perspective. I had a loose primary molar that was hurting so my mom took me to the dentist. He numbed it, removed it, and my pain was gone. That visit made a big impression on me. I knew I could help people and it didn't have to be painful. It was then that I decided I wanted to be a dentist.

I never wavered from that goal and then in 1976, I was married and got accepted to the University of Nebraska Dental School. While in dental school, my wife Carla worked for SRI (now Gallop Inc.). The company developed interviews that could be used to identify the talent and traits needed for success in many different professions. They created one for dental students and then dentists. I was interviewed as a student and that interview was used for training dental school admission's personnel for many years.

Through that connection to SRI, I met the founders of SRI, Dr. Donald Clifton, and Dr. Charles (Chuck) Sorensen, who headed the dental division. Those two men had a profound impact on me as a young man. It was like taking a graduate course in behavioral psychology.

Because Carla worked with Dr. Sorensen, I was fortunate to be invited to attend some of the workshops with other dentists and their staff. They helped me learn how to communicate effectively with my patients and how to utilize the unique talents of each of my staff members.

Armed with my dental degree and great training through SRI, I was eager to practice! I went in with a classmate and we set up a practice from scratch for two new dentists. In hindsight, not the best decision. The economy in 1980 was tough. Our practice loan interest rate was 21%. While we supplemented our income by teaching at the dental school, the practice couldn't support two dentists, so my partner decided to move back to his hometown and work with his father who was also a dentist. I stayed on there to practice for two more years. While the business was building, I still wasn't as busy as I had hoped.

I had a very close friend and classmate who asked me to come join him in Wyoming. The economy there was booming because of the energy industry, and he needed help. I decided to sell my practice and move my young family to Gillette, Wyoming to work with Dr. Larry Bennett in 1985.

As soon as I moved to Wyoming, the oil bust hit. But there was still a solid underlying economy there and the practice grew rapidly. Be careful what you wish for right? I went from a small, slow practice in Lincoln NE, to one that was very busy in Gillette, WY. We had so many patients, but we were frustrated that we couldn't spend the amount of time with patients that we wanted to and that they deserved. The gross income was great, the overhead was high, and the hours were long. It felt like we were losing control of the practice.

We continued to attend SRI seminars with Dr. Sorensen. There I met Dr. Rich Green who was a Cadre member at The Pankey Institute along with other amazing mentors in dentistry. They introduced me to a new level of excellence, comprehensive care, and occlusion principles beyond what I had been taught in dental school. It was Rich who told me about Dr. Michael Schuster who was also Cadre at Pankey. I started following Dr. Schuster through his newsletter, The Profit Letter. It was a newsletter about profitability in dentistry and investments.

When I heard Dr. Schuster was going to be speaking in Denver, Carla and I were excited to attend. At that time, Larry and I had completed two Continuums at Pankey. We loved what we had learned there but were struggling with how to implement it in our busy practices. After listening to Dr. Schuster, I realized I needed business and management training before completing Pankey. I came home and told Larry about what I had learned. We enrolled in the yearlong Management Course at what Dr. Schuster then called the Center for Professional Development.

At the first session, we had a pivotal conversation with Dr. Schuster. He challenged us (as only Mike can) to get our act together. We went back and got to work reorganizing our two separate practices into one sharing everything equally. Larry's wife, Carol, and my wife, Carla both worked in the practice. Together we developed systems and analyzed the numbers. It wasn't always easy, but we were a great team who could discuss things and solve problems together.

That year we experienced immediate improvement. We cut our clinical hours, increased our production, decreased our overhead and our net income went up significantly. The staff size became more manageable, and the staff experienced more ownership and growth. We got control of time and money. Dr. Schuster's percentage budgeting was making a dramatic difference!

It took some time, but we were able to implement many systems like Dr. Schuster's Dental Fitness Program which was an educational tool to give patients objective feedback. It helped them take responsibility for controlling their health. We completed Pankey and refined our new patient process. We used what we learned from SRI for the new patient interview, the Pankey two-appointment model, and with training through the Schuster Center, added "The Dreadful Story" and a printed "Review of Findings" for every new patient.

After a few years, we were working three days a week and six hours a day. At last, we were highly organized, and highly profitable, and our practice was more in line with our values. Although there were always challenges, we were having fun doing high-quality patient care and dentistry. We stayed connected to the Schuster Center via the CEO program and eventually both Larry and I became mentors for other doctors going through the Management Course.

The Schuster Center was about much more than just improving profit. Getting control of time and money allowed us to refocus on professional service and have fun doing it. We actively promoted the Schuster Center in our community and eventually, most of the dentists in Gillette went through the Schuster Center program and The Pankey Institute. I feel like we made a great impact on the quality of dentistry in our community.

Unfortunately, in 1996, I had a freak accident. A glass bottle of apple cider exploded in my hand, cutting the nerves and tendons to my thumb. I tried rehabilitation for a year but with no feeling in my fingers, I never regained proper function or the fine motor skills needed for dentistry. Dentistry had been my passion and was everything I had worked towards since I was 9 years old. Now at age forty-two and in the prime of my career, I lost it all. I was devastated and depressed. I was grieving.

My mission in life has always been to help people and dentistry was my avenue. Eventually, I was able to see that I could still help people. I could help others be prepared for unexpected events. I could help people avoid costly mistakes by planning for their positive dreams and goals. Financial planning was the vehicle I chose – I saw it as "Life Planning".

Using all the training and life lessons I had been so fortunate to experience from the Schuster Center and others, I was able to launch a new career in comprehensive financial planning and wealth management. I realized how I had put the many risk management strategies in place that I had learned from the Center and how needed those were in the financial industry.

I utilize the same philosophy of client intake that I did in my dental practice, only now I am focusing on financial well-being instead of physical health through dentistry. I do believe, however, that financial health has a profound effect on physical and mental health.

After starting with their values and goals, we develop a plan to reduce taxes and incorporate appropriate risk management, debt reduction, and money management. It is their Financial Roadmap – just like the "Review of Findings" I learned from Michael.

The relationships with other dentists from the Schuster Center and the spiritual growth were something I never expected. Meeting other dentists from all over the United States and at different stages of their lives was a tremendous experiential learning process. Those relationships were an education in and of itself. Our friendships are priceless, and we developed relationships that continue to this day.

Dr. Schuster helped me so much as a person and his knowledge, understanding of people and his love for all of us who went through his programs are incredible. The values of the Schuster Center completely matched my values, so it was easy to immerse myself in the philosophy. The Schuster Center stands for treating each person with dignity and respect, and recognizing each person we come in contact with has unique talents and gifts. We have a responsibility to help people.

I will always be indebted to Michael because he challenged me to be a better person and helped me grow and understand my purpose for helping people. Of all the mentors I have worked with, Dr. Schuster had the most profound effect on me, and he continued to support me all these years. I still consider him my mentor, but most of all a wonderful loving friend. I continue to learn from him to this day.

As a side note, I always enjoyed the artistic aspect of restorative dentistry. I believe dentistry is an art form. That love led me to start painting and I now enjoy a career as an artist as well. Michael has been supportive of my artistic endeavors as well.

The following is from www.dingmanwealth.com.

*I grew up in western Nebraska. My father was a farmer, and my mother was a bookkeeper for a local farm implement dealer. As a farm kid, I learned about the value of hard work and that we help our neighbors in times of need. I also learned your crop and future could be wiped out abruptly without warning. I learned at an early age the need for proper risk strategies. I decided to be a dentist and I attended the University of Nebraska and University of Nebraska College of Dentistry. I practiced dentistry in Lincoln, Nebraska, and was a faculty member at the Dental School for two years. My family and I moved to Wyoming, and I practiced dentistry there until I had an accident that ended my career.*

*I attended numerous continuing education experiences that prepared me for staff development, business planning, practice management, and business management. I recognized that a dental school education alone was not going to make me successful. I prepared myself to be the best dentist I could be and developed the necessary business skills to grow my business.*

*I had a life-changing accident. An injury to my right hand caused me to retire from my lifelong passion of being a dentist. Losing my practice was not a pleasant experience, as I saw my business and my dream job in life disappear. Life didn't stop and wait for me to catch up. You never know what lies ahead, however, my life experience and the preparation and education I had sought out prepared me well.*

*I became a financial advisor because I didn't want what happened to me to happen to people just like you. I help people prepare for the ups and downs of life so that they can have a safe and secure retirement.*

# Chapter Twenty-Four
# Dr. Eniko Loud
## Phoenix, Arizona

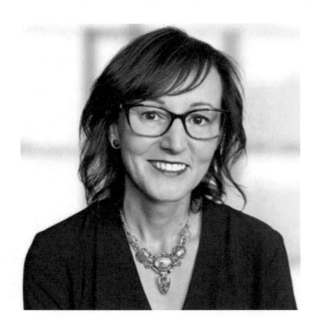

*"I was embedded in the world of name it, blame it and tame it dental disease care. It's a reactive place. Patients take no ownership of their dental conditions. They are insurance-driven and ignorant of the fact that they are on the treadmill of a disease-ridden lifespan. Dr. Schuster gave me the keys to a path that transported me as a person, and my whole practice, toward a new reality. I entered a new dimension, one that I did not know about. In this new world of complete care dentistry, patients collaborate with their doctors and take ownership of their conditions. They get off the treadmill of disease. Together, doctors and patients work toward a common goal of health. It's an empowering way to live in the world. It's a world where I focus on adding and creating value for my patients, my staff, and the world."*

## Growing Up in Romania and Becoming a Dentist

I wanted to be a healer since I was a young child. My mom was a veterinarian and I accompanied her on many home calls. She would explain the physiology of the body, and how it was affected by diseases like cancer. Sometimes I assisted her during surgeries. That early experience awakened my passion for health care and the desire to alleviate people's pain and suffering.

My family lived in Romania, and I enrolled in medical school when I was eighteen years old. During my first year of medical school, I saw several people die from medical mistakes and it soured my desire to become a physician. I learned about dentistry and that seemed like a better fit for me. I'd been artistic growing up with drawing and sculpting. Dentistry seemed like a union of medicine, art, and working with my hands. So, I transferred to dental school in my second year, and I graduated six years later. But I still wasn't sure what I wanted to do. I was going back and forth between medicine and dentistry. So, I went back to school for two more years to finish medical school.

Pursuing the American Dream brought me to the United States. I won the green card lottery, and my application was accepted. My first job was at a 4-H camp in Ohio. Then I went to Cleveland where I worked in a medical lab for three years at minimum wage. I kept moving up the ladder at the lab because I had a strong work ethic, and my English was improving. Then I realized, what the heck am I doing? I have all these degrees that I'm not using. My education was not being applied in my life. I didn't like how the medical system in the US worked, so I explored what it would take to get into dental school. I believed dentistry would give me more freedom to do what I wanted. I was told it's very competitive for foreign-trained dentists, and I would need to score at the 95th percentile on the written boards. Well, I scored 98 and I was admitted into the third-year class at Case Western Dental School. I changed my hours at the lab, and I worked nights so I could attend classes during the day. After graduation, I went into an AGD residency program, and then I worked as an associate for a few professors in their private practices.

I received some good advice from an oral surgeon while I was in dental school. He said, "Figure out where you want to live when you retire and get a license in that state now. Then when you retire, you'll have the freedom to move there and work part-time if you want." I'd been to Arizona on vacation, and I loved it. When my first marriage didn't work out (I got married during dental school) I decided to move to Phoenix, Arizona.

## Startup Practice

I bought a dental practice in Phoenix, but the owner took advantage of me. He made off with most of the patients and erased their records on the computer. I was left with some equipment. So, it was really a startup practice.

Financially, the practice did well, but my time was poorly organized. The practice took over my life and I was working too much. Further, I was taking all types of insurance programs. Previously, I'd worked at a corporate dental office so insurance-driven care was all I knew. I didn't know how to get away from it.

I felt I was just repairing disease. I'm passionate about real health and I realized a lot was missing in the practice. I wanted to get organized around health and healing patients. But I didn't realize what I was doing wrong or how to restructure the practice.

I worked with a popular dental consultant from Oregon, but I was disillusioned with their rigid approach. It was all modeled on the success of a doctor focused on production and repair. Their strategy didn't incorporate my vision and what I wanted to create. Most of the consultants I considered were like that. They didn't integrate the uniqueness of each client with their methods.

I heard about Dr. Schuster at a course in Spain on digital smile design. I was asking lots of questions related to my frustrations and another doctor in the class suggested the Schuster Center could help me. It was destiny! I looked up the Schuster Center online and realized Dr. Schuster was my neighbor, three houses down the street. He was on my neighborhood roster, and I'd even met his wife Patti walking their dog.

I had several goals when I started the Management Program at the Schuster Center including:

- Get out of the insurance business and improve profitability.
- Implement my vision of health and healing. Collaborate with patients to prevent disease and achieve long-term health.
- Slow down and work more reasonable hours.
- Create more time and resources for continuing education in advanced restorative dentistry and holistic health for patients.
- Improve communication and relationships with patients, and effectively implement all the health data I was collecting for patients.

Dr. Schuster helped me face my limitations and my own excuses. I had plenty of them and I needed to move past them.

## Benefits from the Management Year at the Schuster Center

Implementing all the forms and systems to get organized was a lot of work, more than I expected. We had frequent staff meetings and a monthly review of key performance indicators with a Profitability Management Controller Report. My previous consultant did a poor job monitoring our numbers. I had no clue when we were up or down. In fact, working with them my numbers started trending down.

Now we have an office team of eight people. An associate dentist, an office manager, a front desk coordinator, one full-time and one part-time hygienist, and three dental assistants. My staff has been the same with no turnover since I did the Management Program at the Schuster Center.

I quickly recovered my tuition for the Schuster program. I cut back my work hours. I've gone from twenty workdays a month to twelve. Yet, revenue and profit have increased significantly because more patients receive complete care, not just what insurance will cover for the year. It took us three years, but we don't handle insurance anymore. Revenue has increased 20-30% every year since we enrolled at the Schuster Center and collection always equals production. It gives me a big sense of freedom.

We reworked our new patient process, and it was huge. We went from forty to fifty new patients per month down to about fifteen per month. My associate sees some, and I only see five or six new patients myself so I can focus on the patients who want complete care. I brought my associate into the office to care for patients not interested in complete dentistry. Some patients are still loyal to the practice since its inception in 2013 when I was insurance dependent.

Prior to the first new patient appointment, there is a thirty-minute discovery call with the office manager to get acquainted with the patient. I want to ensure the patient is the right fit for our office before they come in.

The new patient appointment is an hour and a half. Instead of just collecting a bunch of data, we restructured the exam to educate patients about preventing disease. We take them through unawareness to awareness of problems. We guide patients through the states of health and give them a Dental Fitness Report card. Patients go home with their plaque and bleeding scores and know where they are on the wellness continuum from sickness (red) to health (green.)

The Review of Findings consult is an hour appointment and occurs about a week later after I get all their reports back. I still use the Pyramid of Health, an educational tool from the Schuster Center for patient consults.

Increased time off allows me to pursue interests I enjoy like learning. I recently completed Level 4 at Orognathic Bioesthetics, Inc. (OBI) a multi-year, advanced restorative dentistry program. Bioesthetic dentistry harmonizes a stable bite with a stable jaw position, healthy comfort and function, and a healthy airway. Now I'm on the faculty track at OBI. It's hard to read dental trade journals after learning the level of excellence taught at OBI.

Prior to OBI, I completed certification in Functional Medicine at the Institute of Functional Medicine (IFM) in Orlando, Florida. It was founded by Dr. Jeffrey Bland at the Cleveland Clinic and Dr. Mark Hyman. Functional Medicine stresses root cause analysis. It's important to me that I understand the whole patient, and that I can work with their physician to optimize their well-being. Certification at IFM is a three to four-year course. I had to submit a written case presentation showing I improved a patient's health and well-being and document the care with lab studies over the course of a year. Certification is valid for ten years, and then I must submit another patient study.

Now I'm studying Ayurvedic Medicine, which looks at disease from a different perspective. Functional medicine looks at causes of disease and healthy physiology, but it's still mostly physical and emotional. Ayurvedic medicine studies subtle forces in the body including the physical, mental, emotional, and spiritual energy of the patient. It takes health to a deeper level than just our physical body. The philosophy behind it is powerful, and it includes the use of diet, herbs, and sensory therapies to balance body systems.

I appreciate the holistic approach of Ayurvedic Medicine, which says the primordial cause of disease is forgetting our true nature, which is spirit, and spirit cannot be ill. We have a lower self and a higher self, and our higher self is our spiritual self. When the lower self can surrender to the higher self, the lower self will experience life through the vision of the higher self, which is spiritual liberation.

Thanks to Dr. Schuster and the Schuster Center I've created a niche, holistic practice, one that marries my interest in medicine with my skills in dentistry. The Schuster model is powerful, and the structure is transformative. I learned from Dr. Schuster that—

*Structure influences behavior and behavior determines results.*

That means it's hard to change behavior unless you change the underlying structure first. Then change in behavior is simple!

For example, prior to the Schuster program, I had structure (policies, organization, and systems) that attracted insurance-driven patients seeking repair dentistry. Now I have practice systems that attract health-centered patients seeking complete, holistic care. It's hard to appreciate the power of structure because it's less visible than behavior. Behavior is the tip of the iceberg that's obvious. Structure is the massive number of beliefs, habits, environment, and more that are under the surface and not seen.

A specific example is the new patient process. Before I had a fast, efficient exam that focused on collecting lots of data about everything wrong with the patient. That allowed me to recommend more treatments and potentially boost production. It's a push strategy with the authoritarian doctor as the expert telling the patient what they need.

Now I slow it down. First, I listen carefully to the patient's goals and concerns with a structured conversation. It's building a doctor-patient relationship. Next, I involve and engage the patient so that they understand and are connected to any problems that hinder their goals. Then together we develop an action plan. It's a collaboration with patient input. It's a pull strategy designed to help the patient want the treatment they need.

The Schuster model was a steppingstone, or really a launching pad that allowed me to create the practice of my dreams. It allowed me to develop my own vision, attract the type of patients I wanted to work with and practice the type of dentistry I enjoy. I haven't done marketing in so long. All our new patients are internal referrals. One patient refers another.

My staff are grateful to be here. They are engaged and we still have regular staff meetings. Of course, they receive raises too. We have the higher goal of health over production and adding value to people's lives. We feel like a family and our love for one another keeps growing. Hearing patients say thank you and receiving gratitude all day long builds a stronger team. It's a positive culture. It's important that my team and my patients are happy to be here.

Recently, I've had thoughts of starting a new practice from scratch where I would do only complete care dentistry. I would see just one patient a day or a few patients a month. But I would be fully involved with all aspects of their care—health coaching combined with Bioesthetic dentistry, Ayurvedic healing, and functional medicine for truly complete health. The sky is the limit now.

*Dr. Eniko Loud received a DDS from the University of Oradea in Romania in 1999. In 2002 she moved to the USA and in 2006 she obtained her DMD from Case Western Reserve University*

*School of Dental Medicine. In addition, she completed an AEGD residency obtaining extensive experience in full-mouth rehabilitation and her mastership degree in implant dentistry. She obtained her Functional Medicine certification in order to provide well-rounded care making her one of three Functional Dental practices in the United States. She completed Level 4 training in advanced restorative training at Orognathic Bioesthetics in 2022. When not in the office, she loves spending time with her husband and her two Vizsla dogs. She practices yoga and enjoys hiking and being outdoors. In 2019 she started Spartan Racing. She believes in challenging herself and achieving goals in her personal life as well as her professional life.*

*Learn more at [https://wholehealthdentistryaz.com/dr-eniko-loud](https://wholehealthdentistryaz.com/dr-eniko-loud)*

# Chapter Twenty-Five
# Dr. Peyton Cunningham

## Shreveport, Louisiana

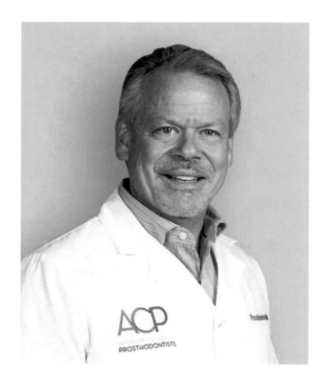

*Over my life, so many doors have opened that I've learned to walk through the door. One door opened for me at the dental lab where I worked in college. Then another door opened when I met Dr. Schuster and attended the Schuster Center. Recently, a door opened for alternative medicine and my personal health. If the door opens, you go in. Don't look back, just do it.*

## Why Dental School?

My family was all into law as a career, but I had no interest in that. I like to build things with my hands, so I started college as a pre-med major. My sophomore year I was on a date with a cute coed, and we ran the car into a tree at sixty miles per hour. I suffered mandibular fractures at the symphysis and both condyles. When I woke up in the hospital, the surgeon about to operate on me was playing the banjo while waiting for the operating room to be ready. I thought a job where you can play the banjo on a break, well that must be a pretty cool job and I better look into it. So, I found a dentist who had an in-house lab. I started waxing up and casting crowns in the summertime before dental school.

I graduated from Louisiana State University Dental School, and then from Prosthodontic Residency at the University of North Carolina Chapel Hill. I earned a master's degree from UNC where I studied stress around dental implants.

## Start-Up Practice – Growth and Struggle

I started my practice from scratch in 1989 in Shreveport, LA. I was the only prosthodontist between Dallas, TX, and Jackson, MS, and from Baton Rouge, LA to Little Rock, AR. I had no training in practice management and no idea how to run a small business. I struggled with staff issues, finding new patients, and paying off my loan. My brother-in-law was a dentist near Shreveport and one Christmas he gave me a book. It was the manual from the Profitability Management Seminar taught by Dr Mike Schuster. My brother-in-law said, "You need to go see this guy." Lo and behold, the manual grabbed me because it was about organization and money, and I didn't have a clue about what I was doing.

I flew to New Orleans with my wife, and we took the Schuster seminar. I was impressed with the course, and I created an Excel spreadsheet to track overhead categories, production, collection, and profitability. It was percentage budgeting according to Dr Schuster's target percentages for overhead, doctor salary, solvency, and return on investment. Soon I took another seminar with Mike and after that, I decided to go out to Scottsdale, AZ for the Management program.

Blair Kolkowski, an analyst for the Schuster Center, came to my office and did a Practice Health Evaluation. It was an assessment of all aspects of the practice, but by that time I was already committed to the Management program no matter what he found. I'm a perfectionist by nature and I needed to know the best way to propose treatment recommendations to patients. Further, I wanted to ensure I was profitable and not wasting money. I needed the structure that the Schuster Center offered to know that I was doing things correctly. The fact that Dr Schuster set a model of what I should aspire to was appealing.

## The Management Program at the Schuster Center – Organization, Control, and Profit

Over the year, my staff and I traveled to Scottsdale three times for a three-day Intensive seminar. Also, I attended a three-day case presentation seminar. I wanted help with all aspects of running a practice. Time control was important. I was busting my butt for patients because I wanted them to get healthy. As a result of that, the practice took over my life. I had a growing family, a wife, and a couple of kids and I needed to have time with them. I was spending too much time in the practice.

Money control was important. I knew how to manage money somewhat, but I wanted to be sure I was putting it in the right places like savings for retirement, new equipment, taxes, etc. I'm frugal and I don't overspend on high-tech stuff. I stick to the percentage budgeting of the Schuster model in the monthly Profitability Management Controller Report. It's like a compass that keeps me on course for the practice financial goals.

Learning to be a leader was important. I didn't know how to manage people, and I lacked leadership skills. I had a revolving door to the office for quite a while until I learned to hire the right people.

Half of my original staff was motivated to learn and apply the policies and systems we created. Staff members who liked structure stayed with the practice, and we saw how the organization benefited the patients and us. I've always had a small office and staff. I worked out of two operatories, and we had a third room for hygiene. I have one hygienist, two dental assistants, and one front office coordinator. My current team has been with me for many years, two for seventeen years, one for seven years, and one for four years.

I had to hire a hygienist after a few years because some cases were so complex the general dentist offices didn't know how to manage them. I needed a hygienist to oversee the periodontal health of those patients. It becomes a real challenge to keep these people healthy because their oral tissues aren't normal. What do you do with a patient who has a full-thickness skin graft from their leg with hair growing out and now that's in their mouth?

My hygienists became very capable to the point where they could change out attachment parts, use implant wrenches, and do other tasks.

I wanted to know how to manage referrals, and where I would get new patients. In the early years, all my patients were referred by other dentists. That changed dramatically over time. In the last twenty years, 70% of patient referrals were from other patients in the practice and 30% were trauma or cancer cases. Occasionally a dentist would call me up and say, "Hey, I can do this case, but I don't want to do it" I thought that was smart because the patient was usually a friend or family relative of the GP, and they had complex dental/facial problems. Those cases take a lot of time, and you have to charge for it, or you will lose money fast.

In dental school, the new patient process is all in pieces, and we think that's the only way. In the Schuster model, Mike consolidated all that, including establishing rapport and trust and engaging the patient with their overall health. It's a struggle to learn at first, but then you just start taking care of the people you can take care of. There are some people who don't want to take responsibility and be helped in that way. I'm trained to do complete dentistry and full mouth restoration when necessary. I know what people need clinically to make treatment work. The Schuster Center gave me the structure and the consultation process, for presenting full-mouth dentistry.

I was trained to do a report of findings in pros school, and I was comfortable presenting large, difficult cases. I was trained in intraoral and extraoral maxillofacial prosthetics, as well as TMD problems. It's not uncommon for people to come in with gunshot wounds to their faces. I go to the operating room with the surgeon and see how we can repair the damage. We use fibula grafts, iliac crest grafts, calverial grafts, and scapular grafts. We put all those bones into the face and the oral cavity. Then we place dental implants and try to get the soft tissue right so that people look well. It's the same with trauma from car wrecks, motorcycle wrecks, boating accidents, or cancerous tumors.

Occasionally I need to do minimal or holding treatment because patients don't make the commitment to move forward with dental restorative treatment. I'm a big proponent of the Dental Fitness Program developed by Mike. After some time in Dental Fitness patients understand the concept of taking control of their health. Then, suddenly they get motivated to complete treatment. It's just phenomenal!

I tracked all new patients and treatment acceptance in the beginning with Schuster Center coaching, and I continued through the Mastery program. I kept monitoring the key indicators, but patients kept coming to the office. Dr Harold Wirth said, "Take care of your patients and they'll take care of you." I did, and patients did, and I never had to worry about new patients after that first year.

Ironically, getting patients healthy with Dental Fitness led to a problem. It demonstrates one of the many mistakes I made. At one point I fired all my hygiene patients, and I wasn't going to have a hygienist anymore. Doctors had stopped referring patients. You see

I was doing Dental Fitness and getting patients healthy. Consequently, they wanted to stay with my office and not their general dentist. I wasn't trying to do that on purpose. I wanted patients to return to their general dentist for periodontal maintenance. However, patients would flatter and pressure my front desk coordinator and work their way into my hygiene schedule. I guess patients could tell which office really had their best interests at heart.

The Management program was a lot of work. In fact, I joke that Mike was a pain in the butt. But he was also very inspiring, motivating, passionate, and caring for those of us who cared about our patients and our team. One night after the first year, I was lying in bed with three to four books from the Schuster Center beside me and I said to my wife, "We should talk about some of this stuff. We just don't know what we don't know."

## Mastery, Performance Coach, and Beyond

After management, I sent Mike a few dozen referrals, maybe more. Many went through Phase One with Mike. No one stayed as long as I did. I was a disciple, and I continued with Mastery, Advanced Case Presentation, and Performance Coach (PC.) I did everything that the Schuster Center offered. I was there for Jacob Needleman and Steven Covey. I did three or four Advanced Case

Presentation Seminars. Our PC group stayed together for ten years, and we still talk with one another. There was just something there that I needed. I know the reasons for that now. It was a personal journey to overcome things that I grew up with. All those courses provided a great opportunity to learn about myself.

Before my training, I made every mistake there is in the book to make. Mastery was a self-discovery process, and that parlayed into the practice. As I developed as a human being the practice became more evolved and more health centered. We helped people achieve their own goals better. It came back with hugs, gifts, and things like that.

For patients with complex problems, I didn't have trouble with case acceptance. I never was insurance dependent. I was fee-for-service from the first day in practice. I didn't discount my fee. I'm not going to do a filling at a lesser cost and go in the hole every time I do it. I never tried to be super-fast and make money on volume. I struggled for a while, but I told patients, "This is what it costs, and this is what I can do."

I think in each one of us who are truly caring, people have an innate sense, and they can feel you care about your patients. You want to make them better, and you're trying to help them. You can learn some of that, but it's already in your aura, in your being. Some people aren't like that. For them, it's show me the money, show me the production, and let me get in more patients.

I've been on staff with the LSU oral surgery department here in town. I don't do many single crowns or fillings. Mostly it's reconstructions. Eventually, I was working so hard that it affected my health. I was a victim of my own success. The better you get at caring for people, then the more people want to see you. I wasn't good at saying no. I tried to slow down as I got older, but people kept coming in with severe damage. I tried working three days a week, but my schedule would go back to four and then five days.

I recently retired at the age of sixty-two. Because of what I learned at the Schuster Center, I had a choice and the financial resources to retire. I have a genetic tendency and a history of cancer in my family. Both my father and brother had cancer. Not long ago, some blood markers were out of the normal range, so I decided to get serious about stress control, and a healthy lifestyle. One of my doctors is trained in Chinese alternative medicine. He helped me understand that cancer is not just genetics. It's also a metabolic issue having to do with my lifestyle and how I take care of myself. Little things can add up over the years.

Over my life, so many doors have opened that I've learned to walk through the door. One door opened for me at the dental lab where I worked in college. Then another door opened when I met Dr Schuster and attended the Schuster Center. Recently, a door opened for alternative medicine and my personal health. If the door opens, you go in. Don't look back, just do it.

I have a plane and I've flown for years. I used to fly to the Schuster Center in Scottsdale for courses. One of my retirement goals is to help Pilots for Patients. We provide free transportation to patients needing medical treatment at major hospitals like the Mayo Clinic, or St Jude's in Nashville.

*Dr. Cunningham has a B.S. degree from Northwestern State University and a DDS from Louisiana State University of New Orleans. He has a Specialty of Dentistry in Prosthodontics and a Master of Science from the University of North Carolina Chapel Hill. He practiced in the Shreveport area for 34 years and was a member of the ADA, Northwest Louisiana Dental Association, Southwest Academy of Restorative Dentistry, American College of Prosthodontists, International Academy of Gnathology, International College of Oral Implantology, River City's Study Group, and the Ark-la-Tex Dental Academy.*

# Chapter Twenty-Six
# Dr. Cree Hamilton

## Las Vegas, Nevada

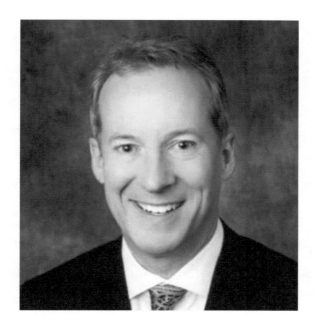

*Almost daily I give thanks for something I have, and I realize Dr. Schuster put that in my life. I wonder what my life would be like if I'd never gone to the Schuster Center. I'd probably be another orthodontist who was successful in the world's eyes, but internally I would be frustrated and disappointed.*

## Why I Chose Dentistry and Specialized in Orthodontics

"I would like you to do something better," my dad said during my senior year of high school. Then he walked away. He was a man of few words.

My dad owned a small business that dealt wholesale auto parts in Wellsburg, West Virginia. He worked long hours all his life. I hung out at the shop growing up and I got all the lousy jobs like cleaning the toilets, counting bolts, and tarring the roof in the summer. I thought I was following in my father's footsteps, and he was teaching me a strong work ethic by making me work my way up from the bottom. I was going to attend college, then come back, work in the shop, and grow the business. Now what would I do?

I found a book describing occupations in the library. I'd had a good experience with my childhood orthodontist, and dentistry seemed attractive. It offered a good living without the life-or-death issues of medicine. I needed to fill out my college application form more than anything. I felt like everybody had their life figured out but me. So, I selected a pre-dental major.

I met two classmates in my dorm who were pre-dental, one of whom is still a close friend. My high school sweetheart and future wife's father was a dental lab technician. When he showed me all the cool equipment he worked with, I was sold on dentistry.

After dental school, I planned to set up practice in my hometown. But I joined the Air Force to get some clinical experience first, make some money, and have fun for three years. The Air Force sent my wife and me to Las Vegas, Nevada. An oral surgeon at Nellis, A.F.B. mentored me and recommended I go into surgery. Surgery wasn't for me. But when my Air Force duty was over, I thought it would be a good time to specialize before getting a loan and starting my own practice. I narrowed my choice down to endodontics or orthodontics. A good friend and dental classmate who went to ortho school right after graduation advised, "Just go ortho and you'll thank me later." So, I returned to West Virginia for ortho school.

After a winter back east, my wife and I decided we wanted to settle in the southwest. I planned to open an orthodontic practice in Las Vegas. I was naïve enough to think I would never fail. I went to all the banks in town requesting a startup loan. I was thinking big, and I wanted a gold-plated practice from the get-go. But I knew very little about business and all the banks turned me down. Finally, an experienced banker counseled me that no bank would risk a loan for what I wanted to do, and I needed to scale it way down. She helped me find a modest office of 1100 square feet, and I bought the part-time practice of the existing orthodontist who was working two days/week with three employees.

I had no business understanding so I visited a few well-known orthodontists in California to learn how they managed their office. In addition, one of my fellow ortho residents had been in general practice for ten years prior to ortho school. I asked him for advice, and he said, "You need to control money, and you need to know people better than you do. Take a Dale Carnegie course for people skills. You don't need to study with Schuster right now. Just take ten percent of all your income and put the money in a separate account. It's a Power account for savings, equipment, taxes, etc. so you can avoid debt, and have money for unexpected expenses." That advice was a huge help to me starting out. I saved ten percent of my income every week, and I subscribed to the Schuster Perspective newsletter.

## Big Volume with Bigger is Better

After attending some practice management lectures, I decided to work with a premier orthodontic consultant at the time. She got me busy following the bigger is the better paradigm. She would compare my production and new starts to other big practices, and it triggered my competitive nature. I was scared to death when she convinced me to sign the lease for an office of five thousand square feet. The practice grew from three employees to a team of fifteen.

I'd been in practice for about six years and the top orthodontists were building Taj Mahal practices. The first topic of conversation at professional meetings was how many new starts you had every month. It felt like a big ego trip. As my practice was growing, I was reading the monthly Schuster Perspective newsletter. I recognized a disconnect between what I was doing in my office and what Dr. Schuster wrote about. He described a smaller-is-a-better-model of practice. I wondered, "Where does it all end? Is it always about more and more production?" Further, we had four children then and my wife was doing all the parenting. I would join family vacations, but I wasn't involved daily.

## The Schuster Model – The Right Fit for my Values

There was a spiritual aspect to Dr Schuster's writing that resonated with my values. I don't believe in coincidences. I haven't experienced the audible voice of God, but I've been nudged along many times over my life. I wasn't desperate, but I started to think there was a better way. I decided to enroll at the Schuster Center after being in practice for seven years. I was open to something different from what I was doing. I knew there was more to dentistry than maximum production.

The first lecture at the Schuster Center by Dr. Schuster was great for the team and me. He explained how money moved through the practice. He said, "Your doctor is going to make money because he's doing the work, because he's the owner, and because he's taking the risk. That's the way it should be. If you don't like that then you can do it yourself. You can go to dental school, take out a big loan, open a practice and the buck can stop with you." I had never fully realized that in my own mind. I thought, hey, I deserve to make some money.

I'm not a numbers guy, and tracking money in the practice doesn't do much for me. But I learned I had to do it, and we got better control of money. Then I trained a capable assistant and delegated it.

I started as a micromanager in practice, but I'm more of a big-picture guy. I painted the vision and values for the practice and delegated the rest. That suits me better. Dr Schuster helped me with that. He told me, "What are your values? Write them down and then live them. Make a vision and then develop policies and systems that follow that."

That was dramatically different from what the orthodontic consultants advised. They told me how to be efficient for maximum production. I made money but I was stressed and unbalanced. Dr.

Schuster gave me a strategy to figure out what I should be doing to align my work life with my own values. I discovered how to be effective, provide good orthodontic treatment, have fun, and earn a fair profit.

Getting control of money enables all the other aspects of management, like controlling time, getting organized, and determining the types of procedures you enjoy doing and the types of patients you enjoy treating. Of course, the joke is that orthodontists don't really do anything, that we delegate everything and then just show up.

Almost daily I give thanks for something I have, and I realize Dr. Schuster put that in my life. I wonder what my life would be like if I'd never gone to the Schuster Center. I'd probably be another orthodontist who was successful in the world's eyes, but internally I would be frustrated and miserable. Next to my father and paternal grandfather, Dr. Schuster has had the most influence on my life. Much of that influence was early in our relationship, but the people he introduced me to, the philosophies, and the books were transformative.

The change started with getting control of money and time. Then came team development. I never had much staff turnover. Many of my employees have been with me for over twenty years.

Some of them were mentors to me. If you're open to learning, and listening to people, and you use discernment according to your values, everyone can be a resource.

I wanted to hire people who had skills to make up for my deficiencies. That was huge for me. I had to let go of my ego. I learned if people love and trust you, they will be a better ambassador for you than you can be for yourself. It got to the point where people came in saying how much they had heard about me. I was almost afraid to meet them because I didn't want to disappoint them. I don't need a reputation as Superman. I just need people to love and respect me.

I had more time off, and less stress, I was not on any insurance plans, and I had professional freedom. I wasn't chained to the chair four days a week, and I had time and money to take vacations. I took advanced training at Roth Williams School, the Kois Institute, and Spear. Whenever I took a CE workshop, I took off the day before and the day after classes, so I had time to go over my notes and develop a strategy for what I'd learned.

My practice continued to grow for the next ten years. I was still trying to rationalize that bigger is better. Living in Las Vegas is crazy. Everyone is trying to keep up with the Joneses. I've heard it said, it's hard to live in the world and not be of the world. But I didn't want to keep growing. I was still listening to Dr. Schuster regularly and connected to the Schuster Center with the Performance Coach program.

I took Dale Carnegie classes twice, then I assisted, and then I went through instructor training. I taught a fourteen-week class for two years with forty students in the class. That was invaluable. But it was a big eye-opener in Performance Coach when we had to take videos of our consultations. I hated looking at the videos. You don't need feedback from a consultant when you watch yourself. The video shows every flaw, and you see it yourself. I realized most of the magic happened when I left the room and the treatment coordinator patched things up. The only saving grace was there were a few dentists at the training who were worse than I was. It took some heat off me, but I had no illusion that I was good.

I went back and worked on consults with my treatment coordinator, who had lots of dental experience. I asked her to give me feedback immediately after every new patient. After I was done, she'd come in and say "You were doing so good, and then you went off on a tangent and you said blah, blah, blah. I could see the patient lose interest. You didn't need to say that." I said, "OK good point, thanks." Or she would say "You said uhm thirty-seven times." And I said, "uhm."

My classmates at the Schuster Center recognize the difficult work we did. It's easy to be critical of the world and blame external forces for our problems but it's so difficult to look within ourselves. I remember one day Dr. Schuster metaphorically grabbed me in the hall and shook me. He said, "What the hell are you doing? You hear all this stuff, and you repeat all this stuff. Does your practice and life reflect all this?" So, I spent a good year asking myself if I had integrity in what I said and what I did. If somebody doesn't love you, they won't confront you like that.

## Getting Serious About Slowing Down and Living with Integrity

In 2005 I fired all my consultants. I'd been in practice for sixteen years, and I wanted to really slow down. Dr. Schuster talks about integrity from a sense of being whole or a "wholistic" approach to talking to patients and spending time with them. I'd always rationalized that orthodontists don't do that. Rather, it's transactional, one chair to another. Let the staff schmooze all the people because they like doing it and they're so much better at it than I am. But that was a cop-out. I became more authentic, and I didn't have to be a different person going to work than I was outside the office. If I wanted to give someone a hug, I'd do it. If I wanted to say, "God bless you," I just did it and let the chips fall where they may.

Also, in 2005 I decided I wasn't going to work more than 144 days a year, or twelve days per month. When my associate came in a few years later I decreased to 10.5 workdays per month. I was getting older, and I enjoyed having time to talk with patients. Relationships with the team, patients, family, and friends became the higher priority. My quality of life and enjoying every day was more important than increasing income. I had financial security, but I wanted less stress and more peace of mind.

I stopped doing procedures that I didn't love, and I stopped working hours that I didn't want to be in the office. Further, I stopped working with unpleasant patients. I got them to a stable point in treatment and moved them along to someone who could handle them better than me. I stopped trying to get along with difficult team members and helped them find an office where they were a better fit.

I progressively reduced time with dental politics and the local dental society. Initially, I was actively involved, and I did a good job. But It's not my favorite activity and I'm happy with my small circle of influence. I kept eliminating stressors in my life and practice until I got to the point where I loved coming to work every day. I would leave the office saying to myself, hey, today was a good day! Even the bad days are pretty darn good. If you treat people you love, you work with a team you love, you do procedures you love, and you get paid for it, then what's not to like?

I do an annual men's retreat up on the mountain for my church. Earlier I brought together some strong spiritual men so we could do father and son activities together. For three years I facilitated an authentic manhood community. I learned many men don't have close male friends, especially when they need help in a crisis or when they feel disabled. It's important to have a friend for that, and for someone who will call out your blind spots, like when you say one thing but do something else. That's what my fellow mentors in Performance Coach are for me. I believe Performance Coach was initially set up to work 80% on your practice and 20% on your life, but our group works 80% on our life and 20% on our practice. Maybe that's just the way our group worked out.

The books Dr. Schuster exposed us to are especially helpful. One was a book on Transitions by Bridges. Two years ago, I cut back to eight workdays a month. I needed the extra open time as I'm not as sharp or as fast as I used to be. I'm still working on figuring out my semi-retirement. I don't want to jump into the next thing too fast. I learned it can take a year or more to go through that transition and find your new legs.

## Transitions – The Future

I tell young people there are thirty-one Proverbs in the Bible like there are often 31 days in a month. Get The Message version of the Bible and take five minutes a day to read the Proverb corresponding to that day. King Solomon was the wisest and richest man that ever lived. Even if you don't believe in the Bible, history supports those two statements. He wasn't perfect but there's a lot of wisdom there. It's helped me stay out of a lot of trouble.

I'd like to have a plan for moving forward. Dr. Schuster often says, "You can do anything you want, you just can't do everything you want, so get really clear." There's a saying about where to put your energy to be happy, i.e., to have, to do, or to be. I'm a doer, a performer, but I'd like to just be present in my life more. I've accepted that enough is enough. I don't need to have my voice heard, or my practice numbers be at the top to placate my ego. I prefer spending time with my family and a few close friends. I'll have no problem if my partner takes my name off the building when I fully retire and leave the office.

At one time my office was geared toward high volume, the traditional orthodontic model. Now, the biggest difference you would notice between my office and other orthodontists in town is volume. Most offices see about one hundred patients a day. We see half that number between two orthodontists. I've tried to be both high-tech and high-touch, but over the last decade, I've put more emphasis on the high-touch aspect and building relationships with patients and team members.

Occasionally patients will comment that our fees are higher. I take that opportunity to share that when I began my practice, I had to make some decisions. I decided that I wanted to work in a comfortable and pleasing environment where I would enjoy treating family and friends, and have access to the best materials, equipment, technology, and continuing education. Two more things were vitally important. One, I did not want to be in a position where insurance companies could dictate what type of treatment I rendered. Two, I wanted to hire and train the best team possible. This all costs more money, but I have been blessed that our patients have discovered a greater value here than finding it cheaper somewhere else.

Although we have higher fees, we try to make it affordable and remove financial barriers to patients starting treatment. Because orthodontics usually takes twelve months or longer, we provide in-house financing at no interest. We run credit checks and extend credit accordingly. If people choose in-office financing, we have them sign an ACH for their monthly payment. It increases our odds of collection over requesting a check for their monthly payment.

I found it's important to have great systems to make everything work. If a patient falls behind in their payment schedule, then our doctor-patient relationship declines. They start picking apart my dental work because they need to somehow validate not paying me. Today that means poor online reviews and a lot of damage control to get them back into the relationship. Sometimes it means sticking to my guns if they have a poor credit score and having them pay 50% upfront, and the second 50% over the first half of the treatment time.

I've done some mentoring for dentists. What I enjoy now is seeing my business partner take what I've learned, and what he's learned, and use the creative process to grow and develop his practice and his life. After working here a few years he went from associate status to partner. He's a full partner now and he makes the management decisions and controls operations in the practice. He's a natural leader. I was delighted when he said to me, "I don't want a satellite office anymore. I just want to work twelve days a month like you. And if we could work together on some of those days that would be great too." Wow, he gets it! He wants to be available for family time and a balanced life. Well done!

*https://www.hamiltonortho.com/meet-your-orthodontists/*

# Chapter Twenty-Seven
# Dr. Scott McKinney
## McLean, Virginia

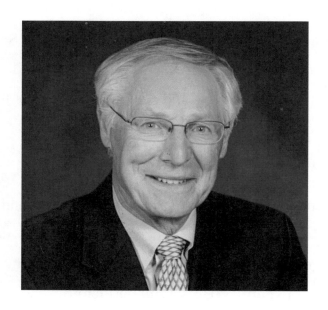

*"I came to the Schuster Center for help merging three practices with different philosophies. I was burned out and brain dead. My future looked dark. I soon discovered my initial idea was not what I wanted at all.*

*The Schuster Center changed my life. It allowed me to focus on being me. Until you get control of money you never become the person you want to be.*

*The Schuster Center is like the Yellow Brick Road in the Wizard of Oz— the proverbial path to the land of your hopes and dreams. It represents strategy, how you will get there, and the best and smartest way to accomplish your goal."*

## Why Dental School

I was ten years old when I won a lawn mower in a raffle at a local gas station. My working-class dad encouraged me to become an entrepreneur. He said, "Scott, why don't you start a business." I liked that idea, and I asked around the neighborhood for customers. I got a job mowing the lawn of a dental office (in a house) two houses away.

One day while Dr. Jack Carroll was taking a smoke break on the office back porch he asked me, "Scott, what are you going to do when you grow up?" I hadn't really thought beyond my lawn-mowing business. He took me into his office and showed me some X-rays, plaster models of teeth, and his dental equipment. He explained how he filled a cavity and fixed broken teeth. I liked building model airplanes; some I even flew. In dentistry, I could build things. That day he planted the seed of a dental career in my mind. Dr. Carroll paid my first-semester tuition at Georgetown University School of Dentistry, September of 1968.

I was the first one in my family to go to college. I attended a small, liberal arts school, Franklin College, in Indiana, and I chose Biology, a pre-dental major. The neighborhood dentist wrote a letter of recommendation for me when I applied to dental school. After graduation, I was accepted to Indiana Medical/Dental School and

Georgetown Dental School. I chose dentistry because medicine seemed like it would take up too much of my life. I joined the Navy Reserves as a freshman in dental school because I wanted to have a job and gain clinical experience when I graduated.

One experience at Georgetown dental school is memorable. It foreshadowed my deep dive into TMD therapy for the second half of my dental career. I had become friends with Dr. Peter Neff. He taught occlusion and was an alumnus of the Pankey Institute. Dr. Neff used to meet occasionally with Pete Dawson and Charlie Stuart (two renown restorative dentists) to discuss centric relation or stable jaw position.

One session Dr. Neff allowed me in the conference room to observe. I remember they screamed at one another the entire time over the definition of Centric Relation. Finally, Dr. Neff said to me, "You mister, up against the wall. Now relax your jaw" With his hand guiding my chin he said, "Forward and back, forward and back." Then he strongly shoved my mandible and head as far back as they would go. He turned to the others and said, "That's CR!"

When the meeting was over, I went up to Dr. Neff and said, "Dr. Neff I don't know much about occlusion, but if that's CR I know I don't ever want it."

## Distress Over Finances and Working in Multiple Offices

After my tour in the Navy, I started a group practice from scratch in Arlington, VA with two professors from school. We each borrowed $25,000 to get started and we remodeled the office suite ourselves. I taught at the dental school one day a week in oral diagnosis and treatment planning. The practice got busy quickly and we even brought in an associate at a satellite office.

Seven years later we started having problems. It seemed like we were all just bouncing around and going nowhere. My two partners had little concern for the profitability of the practice. They received fixed income from full-time teaching positions at the dental school. I heard Dr. Mike Schuster's lecture at a seminar in 1979, and I felt we needed to get better organized and more profitable. I knew of Mike from other dentists and from instructors at school. Some were faculty at the Pankey Institute in Florida where Mike was also faculty. I had all of Mike's books and tapes. My push for organization and getting control of money caused friction with my partners.

Then it got more complicated! Eventually, I was renting space in one office, working part-time in the group practice, building a new office in McLean, VA, and helping a family in another office where the father, an older dentist had been killed in a car accident. The family wanted me to buy the practice. Then, tragically, one of my partners in my group practice was killed in an automobile accident. Our accountant called me. I had stopped working there, but my name was still on the lease, and I was legally responsible for everything done by the associate and bills. Is your head spinning yet? I know mine was! I had multiple offices in different locations, and it was a total mess.

At ten o'clock one night, after a full day on the treadmill of my life, I stopped at the traffic light two miles from home, and I had a panic attack. I just started shaking uncontrollably. I went home and told my wife Betsy (my soul mate, who I met in the fifth grade) I couldn't do it anymore. I enjoyed my patients, but my frantic, scattered work life was a recipe for disaster. We talked and I decided to consolidate two offices into the new office building in McLean and sell or back out of everything else.

McLean is eight miles from the White House, an affluent community, home to many diplomats, military, members of Congress, high-ranking government officials, educated people with wonderful families, "beltway bandits" and seniors. I made connections in the community by living there, and the practice quickly got busy. Patients wanted ideal treatment like I had been taught in school and insurance restrictions were not an issue. I hired an associate right away, and then we expanded the office space to accommodate another young dentist who had lost his lease. The office went from 2,500 square feet to 5,000 square feet.

In a few years, I had over 2,500 active patients, an associate, three full-time hygienists, two assistants, and two front desk staffers, for a combined staff of sixteen people. I shared space with the third dentist who had moved in when we expanded. He had his own staff. Both my associate and I worked five days a week. We had good revenue, but I wasn't making any money. I had a practice loan, and any money that came in was immediately spent. We had no control of money or time, and we had no structure or organization. It was crazy. Our overhead was around 62-72% and I wasn't saving any money.

I loved clinical dentistry, but I knew we needed help. Practice management in school had been a one-hour class, and, of course, there was no practice management in the Navy. The two younger dentists wanted to form a partnership. I told them the only way I would consider it was if we all went through the Schuster Center first.

## Schuster Center Management Program

So, we enrolled in the Management program, and I flew our combined staff of sixteen people out to Scottsdale, AZ three times over the next year. At the first session, Dr. Schuster met with the three dentists and we each had a turn explaining our expectations for the future. As mentioned previously, the two young dentists wanted to form a partnership. I was reluctant and I wasn't sure it was the best option for all of us. Dr. Schuster advised that we postpone a decision and revisit the issue after completing the management program.

My goals for the Schuster Management Program were to improve profitability, get control of money and time, get organized, and determine if a partnership made good sense. Ultimately, the dentists all went their own ways, but I continued to have an associate.

The practice became more profitable, and we got organized. At the end of the year, I had $120,000 in the bank! I'd never had cash in the bank my entire life. I paid off the $60,000 tuition for the Schuster program and still had $60,000 left over sitting in the bank. I learned the difference between wealth and income. Income (or production) is ego. Wealth (net worth) is financial freedom and independence. I got the magic of compounding working for me with savings (solvency and ROI accounts) instead of working against me with debt and loans.

I started doing a two-appointment examination and Review of Findings consultation while in the Management Program. Patients would comment, "Nobody ever spent this much time with me." There was a clear separation between my practice and other dentists in town. It led to a boost in patient loyalty and trust in our office, as well as patient referrals of their friends, family, and co-workers.

I didn't know these things previously, but now it all makes sense. Patients were informed, they could see problems and what was happening in their mouth, and they made their choice for treatment based on facts. We had some wonderful patients who were very successful in their careers. It was easy to present or promote good dentistry, and I believed I was doing the right thing for people.

Even though they were skeptical and frightened initially, my staff became believers in what we were doing. They had input into the changes and the policies and systems we implemented. Since then, I've had very little staff turnover. Most of my employees have been here for twenty-five years or more.

## Mastery Program

A few years later I continued study at the Schuster in the two-year Mastery program. I did it because I could. I'd experienced first-hand the benefits of the Schuster model. With time and money under control, I could take time out of the office to work on my practice and myself. I had time for family, for serious, hands-on continuing education, and for recreation. I was able to coach Little League baseball for thirteen years.

Mastery helped me refine my vision and purpose in the direction I wanted to go. I prioritized the procedures I enjoyed the most, and the patients I felt most able to help. Further, I enjoyed the health and wellness aspect of Mastery, as well as the coaching around leadership, communication, and relationship building. Betsy also appreciated the course material, and we shared many good books with hours of reflection. She was a dental hygienist, office manager, mother, and life partner. We developed a one-year, a five-year, and a ten-year life plan and financial plan. We learned that when expectations are not defined, then frustration and disappointment are certain. Benefits from planning together spilled over into our lives outside of the office.

Managing transitions was a study topic from Mastery (see Transitions, by William Bridges.) Part of that curriculum was the phrase, "Act as if and you will become it." This statement had a profound influence on me. It takes the present and projects it into the future. It required me to consciously act as though I had already achieved my goal, even though I might doubt my ability or face daunting challenges.

If I want to be healthy, the only way I can be healthy tomorrow is to act healthy today. If I want to be wealthy tomorrow, then today I must start doing what wealthy people do. If I continue to "act as if" what I wish to become, eventually it happens. This is what I think spiritual mentors mean when they write about "beingness. I can't be a certain way until I act that way. I became more aware, analytical, and determined. I might think or talk a certain way, but I could not "be" a certain way until I acted the same way I dreamed (my vision) of becoming.

I came to understand I was the activating force! Yes, I was the force behind change in my practice and lifestyle. The only thing I can change is what I'm doing now. I became fully focused. It's like golf where I choose my club, commit to the choice, and execute the swing. I supplied energy, developed a plan, and executed the plan. The only thing I can control is what I'm doing now. I can't change or control the past. I must look beyond it. I can't live in the future, but I can envision one. The actions I take now shape the future I'm creating. I can't control the past or the future. I can only live in the present.

As a result of my Center experience, I acted "Act as if" twice. Once when I realigned the practice financial aspects to conform with the Center's Model. That action resulted in the second. I limited my practice to TMD-related patients, difficult restorative cases, studying, teaching, and lecturing locally and nationally for OBI, Orognathic Bioesthetics, International.

Five years after enrolling at the Schuster Center, the proof was in the numbers. Everybody in the office was making more money. In 1999 I gave a presentation at the Schuster Center Annual Learning Conference titled, *It Wasn't Always Like This: A Way to Profitability, Emotional Maturity, and Peace.* I shared spreadsheets of key performance indicators before, during, and after working with the Schuster Center team. It was a thorough statistical analysis of my practice production, collection, overhead, outcomes, and shortfalls. The financial numbers of the practice for five consecutive years were open for all to see, scrutinize, and question.

The presentation also included published statements by staff members. It was not just about numbers and statistics. People's lives and livelihoods could be deeply affected. There was a lot of genuine soul-searching. At the conclusion of the presentation my staff and I answered questions from the audience. We wanted to share our experience honestly and openly with other offices, both doctors and staff. We hoped to address concerns of "How to do it," and "What if," and make the journey less intimidating.

Here is some of what I presented:

*I came to the Schuster Center trying to find a way to combine three practices and deal with differing philosophies and widely divergent personalities. I wanted to organize all the operations with proven business principles.*

*I was burned out and brain-dead. I could not even react. The future was dark. After the first session of Management, I knew what I contemplated doing was not what I wanted at all. The further we went during Management the more clearly I saw what I really wanted. I found the practice model that was a better fit and decided what was necessary.*

*The old system created the problem. The concept of what I was doing was to get away from the ME (separateness of the parts,) and into a WE (parts make the whole). The better the whole did the better the parts did - each part was a required component of the whole but could not function independently of the whole.*

*I found that my overhead was high, specifically in the labor category. Modifying that resulted in sweeping rewards. I rehired everyone in the practice reducing the labor/collection ratio to conform with the Schuster Model. I engaged the workers in an honest discussion of both the cost and quality of work that is needed for the business to thrive.*

361

*I informed, involved, and empowered all the team members. I let them understand the situation and collectively influence the practice structures.*

*The changes I/we made are life changing. They affected my team members, my wife, and myself. It's not the only way, but it's a way that worked for us. Mutual respect, hard work, and open communication have been foundational in our success efforts.*

My presentation focused on getting control of money. I wasn't living beyond my means, but I wasn't saving any money. Dr. Schuster said, "The first step of any successful practice is to get control of money. To put systems and strategies, at whatever cost, at whatever price, in place to control the flow of the resource."

I believe the numbers speak for themselves. The team worked for it and we did it working fewer days. We never looked back. Every following year was easier and better. We all became better people for it.

- Collections increased 18%.

- Overhead decreased by 8%, from 62% previously to 54% after.

- Savings in solvency accounts increased from 0 to 10%.

- Return on investment (ROI) increased from 0 to 10%.

- Additional profit shared with the team increased from 0 to 5%.

Was I afraid? Yes, I was. But I was more frightened by the thought of not being able to provide for our retirement. Further, I was frightened of not having some days off, or worse, not having good health to enjoy my retirement. That was being afraid!

## Advanced Clinical Training, Practice Refinement, and Teaching

After completing Mastery Dr. Schuster recommended that I get more clinical training in restorative dentistry. So, I enrolled in Orognathic Bioesthetics, International. I had always wanted to learn more about TMD and occlusion since watching Doctors Neff, Dawson, and Stuart debate in dental school (all published books and articles.) After completing OBI, I felt prepared to treat difficult, complex cases. I hosted a dinner, and I invited thirty dental colleagues from my sphere of influence, general dentists and specialists. I gave a presentation showing how I could help them treat some of their difficult patients.

I soon had more patients than I could handle because few dentists knew how to handle TMD, surgical cases, and complex occlusion problems. I developed a close relationship with Dr. Joe Mauro, an outstanding oral surgeon in Michigan who I met through OBI. I traveled to Michigan at least a dozen times to assist Dr. Mauro in the OR with my patients who had orthognathic surgery. I could afford to do it, and I wanted to give the best support and care to my patients.

So, I retired from doing general dentistry to focus solely on TMD treatment and people with occlusal problems. When I stopped doing general dentistry, patients cried. But I still got to see them in the office. I was off in one operatory. The rest of the office carried on as usual, but I was away from the hustle and bustle.

Eventually, I sold the practice to a retired Navy dentist. He couldn't believe how well the office ran on its own. He flourished and he could focus on the clinical care of patients. All the staff who had been through the Schuster Center program stayed with the practice. I joined the OBI faculty and became active in teaching with Dr. Jeff McClendon and a few others. I loved the teaching and the type of dentistry I was doing. I continued with that for almost twenty years. One year I was on the road teaching so often I was only home for two weekends. Fortunately, my wife Betsy was supportive. She recognized I had a special calling for the work.

I developed relationships with some wonderful people, leading TMD dentists, restorative dentists, specialists, and researchers. We would discuss new knowledge and learn from one another. It was very stimulating and satisfying. I even became an expert witness in jury trials. I would see Dr. Neff and Dr. Dawson annually at the American Equilibration Society meeting. I'd thank them and we'd laugh about the early days.

I got to spend time with Sam Queen, a research biochemist who came to Washington DC to testify before Congress. We became friends. Betsy and I spent lots of personal time with him. Sam developed Free Radical Therapy which promotes health at the cellular level. Cellular health of the TMJ is critical, and it became an integral part of my therapy for patients.

## The Proverbial Path to the Promised Land of One's Hopes and Dreams

Once while giving a lecture to dentists, I made an offhand comment that the Schuster Center was like the yellow brick road in The Wizard of Oz. A doctor asked me what I meant by that. I decided to think it through and write down how the Schuster Center was like the yellow brick road.

*The Yellow Brick Road in The Wizard of Oz represents strategy, how you will get there, and the path you identify as the best and smartest way to accomplish your goal.*

- *Dorothy is you, the dentist. The protagonist in confusion and turmoil, looking for a vision, a way out, to self-actualization or the realization or fulfillment of one's talents and potential.*

- *The Scarecrow is your brain. Your effort to learn and study; understand the present and the possibilities.*

- *The Tin Man is your heart. It's your will or spirit, your determination.*

- *The Lion is your courage. It's your commitment required to undertake the journey through the unknown. Your ability to counter fear and challenge of the unknown, as well as the difficulties of future change.*

- *The Wizard (Oz) is Dr. Schuster and the Center team, the all-knowing mediators, or messengers of spiritual profundity. The Center is a great depth of knowledge and understanding that supports the process of self-actualization or the grasping of the goal by revealing the power that was always within the student. "The great and powerful Oz*

366

*knows why you have come. The beneficent Oz has every intention of granting your request. But first, you must prove yourself worthy by performing a very small task. Bring me the broomstick of the wicked witch of the West." (Obtaining the broomstick: just put everything as you know it at risk – a very small task?)*

- *Your Brain, Heart, and Courage are virtues needed to find "Home," to discover yourself, the person and place you want to be. If you commit and act on the information presented and guided by the Wizard, you will discover that you alone have within you - your power - to achieve what you want. The struggle is worth the reward. What you seek is within you already.*

# Chapter Twenty-Eight
# Dr. Timothy Leary
## Menlo Park, California

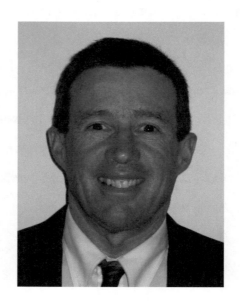

*We spent three years at the Schuster Center, starting with a year in the Management Program, focused on financial growth through time management, money control, and organizing systems and strategies. The second year, part of the Mastery Program, centered on emotional growth by enhancing relationships, leadership, and communication, often referred to as EQ. This empowered both the doctor and the dental team. The final year emphasized spiritual growth, refining our purpose and recognizing the practice's role in serving patients' best interests, aligning our work with our core values and renewing our energy.*

## Startup and Growth

If I compare how I started in dentistry to how I ended up, I realize there was a big transformation. I wandered in the forest for several years before I found the right wizard and the right magic to help slay the dragons. There were multiple dragons in my life: the insurance dragon, the staff management dragon, the single tooth repair dragon, the treatment rejection dragon, and the faster is better, high volume, aerobic dentistry dragon. The magic to slay the dragons was a slower, health-centered model, and offering comprehensive care to patients. Now, my motto is '*Go Slow to Go Fast.*' The magic helped my patients achieve better oral health. Further, it helped me, and my team find more financial and emotional rewards, more fun, and more meaningful work.

I graduated from dental school at the University of Pacific in California. Then, I did a one-year general practice residency in the Air Force in Tucson, AZ. Subsequently, I served in the Air Force Dental Corps for three years. The Air Force experience helped with my confidence, and with my clinical skills when I entered private practice.

After discharge from the Air Force, I took a job as an associate in a busy family practice. I built up my associate practice by being a jack-of-all-trades. I was able to perform some specialty procedures like endodontics, and third molar extractions with IV sedation. Previously the owner's dentist had referred those procedures to specialists. Further, it helped that I enjoyed treating children. In dental school I was told, to do a good job treating her children and mom will become a patient. Take good care of Mom and then Dad eventually makes his way into the office. Also, I took 2-3 times the required amount of continuing education. Patients told me I was friendly and gave a painless injection. In four years, my associate practice was big enough that I needed a hygienist two days a week.

## Limited Success, But Frustration with Production Based, Repair Dentistry

After five years as an associate, I bought a well-established practice in the same building and immediately had a busy practice of 2500 patients. It was an insurance-driven, production-driven, hygiene-driven, family practice. I had two hygienists every day, and three on one day. It was aerobic dentistry running from room to room checking hygiene patients and working out of 2-to 3 treatment rooms with two dental assistants. Practice management taught by the Pride Institute was the biggest influence on me then. The custom of splitting appointments into doctor time and assistant time was popular with experts on the lecture circuit. The goal was to maximize efficiency so that the doctor was always chairside with a spinning handpiece. Everything reversible was delegated to auxiliaries.

Financially I did well, but it was often frantic and high stress. One emergency, an impression to redo, or a crown cementation needing several adjustments would cause a cascade of being late for subsequent appointments. It was professionally frustrating because it was single tooth, repair dentistry made to fit into insurance restrictions and calendar year limits.

I started doing a written Review of Exam Findings (ROFs) for new patients. It made sense to document what I discovered during an exam. It organized my thinking, provided medical-legal protection, and gave the patient time to understand and process any problems. I learned about the ROFs from a tape series by Mike Schuster titled, *Developing and Managing a Practice for Excellence*. Patients liked the non-technical report and personalized treatment plan. They were impressed that I took the time to document everything covered during their exam. The ROFs generated more new patient referrals than anything I had ever done, and it promoted substantial practice growth.

So, I got even busier. I added an associate working 2-3 days/week. I had a team of eleven employees with five part-time hygienists, two dental assistants, one rover, and two front office coordinators. I had a full-time administrative person who filed and followed up on insurance claims. She really worked for the insurance companies, but I paid her salary. It was a massive effort just trying to organize a staff meeting due to all the part-time hygienists working in different offices on various days of the week.

## Learning A New Paradigm

I heard Dr. Schuster speak at a one-day seminar in San Francisco. He described a style of practice that made more sense to me. It was more professional, less stressful, and still profitable. After a Practice Health Evaluation (PHE) I decided to enroll in the one-year practice development program, and my goals were:

- Become less dependent on insurance-driven care.
- Decrease stress, jumping around between multiple treatment rooms and checking hygiene patients.
- Improve team dynamics and boost morale.
- Determine the feasibility of bringing in my associate as a partner.

Schuster Center coaching helped me clarify how I wanted to practice. Then, they got me organized with written systems and protocols around that vision. My practice was transformed from repair dentistry to health-centered care. It was exciting right from the first class. There was a logical, stepwise process so that we could build on one improvement after another. First, was getting financial control with percentage budgeting and Key Performance Indicators. We reviewed the practice numbers monthly with a Profitability Management Controller Report (PMCR.) I came to appreciate the principle, *what gets measured gets done*. Staff helped me create written policies and systems to document administrative operations, and to control overhead.

Second was controlling stress and busy work with patient qualification, and block scheduling. Patient qualification meant targeting the patients who were the right fit for the practice. We designed an experience and an office to attract those patients. Block scheduling meant pre-booking the schedule for the type of dentistry I enjoyed doing. Getting control of time and the appointment book was wonderful! I learned that nearly 80% of the practice profit came from 20% of the patients in the practice. Those were the patients who accepted my recommendations for long-term solutions and complete dentistry. Four months after starting the program I had recovered the full year of tuition.

Next, I refined how I wanted to work, and the type of dentistry I preferred doing. I knew I wanted to slow down, see one patient at a time, and see every patient on time. Further, I wanted to focus on prevention, optimal oral health, and comprehensive treatment.

I worked on improving the new patient process, and the change was phenomenal! We made the new patient exam into two appointments. The first appointment was designed to involve the patient in co-discovery, co-diagnosis, and prevention to avoid dental treatment. The second visit, a week later, was a half-hour consultation with the written Review of Findings. It included facial and intra-oral photographs to review problems and treatment options.

The revised new patient experience was more effective in attracting the right patients and building trust in our office. It led to increased acceptance of complete dentistry. Patients wanted the treatment they needed to get healthy, NOT just what insurance would pay for that year.

Previously, I had no idea of the power of this process. Consultants and lecture experts recommended efficiently collecting exam data and giving patients a treatment plan at the first visit. Some advocated that staff perform parts of the exam. The incorrect belief pervasive in dentistry was that patients would not return for a second consultation visit. My experience showed that was wrong. Why would I rush an incredible opportunity for internal marketing with a prospective client for comprehensive care?

With two appointments I could slow down and discuss the

patient's goals, engage them in the exam, and begin relationship building. In addition, the office was becoming a learning lab. We tracked what treatment patients accepted or rejected, which helped me develop better consultation skills. It's easy for patients to accept limited treatment covered by insurance benefits—somebody else is paying the bill. It's significantly different when patients accept elective treatment and pay out of their own wallets.

We finished up the Management year focusing on team dynamics so that staff was fully trained, confident, and empowered to manage their own departments.

## Transformation with Mastery

Because of excellent progress during the first year, I continued with Schuster Center support in a program called Mastery. Delta, the largest PPO in CA had recently announced they were dropping the highest reimbursement rate from 90% to the 80th percentile. So, I set the goal to drop out of Delta and to stop taking the assignment of benefits from insurance companies. I wanted support from the Schuster Center during that time to minimize patients leaving the practice.

A unique aspect of the Mastery program was called "the Doctor as a model of health." So, in addition to practice development and professional goals, I participated in a wellness program. I set goals for personal health regarding exercise, diet, stress control, oral health, and family/recreation time. Every six months I had my blood chemistry evaluated, I had a stress EKG, and I submitted a three-day diet diary. It was an excellent learning experience and helped me appreciate what a patient goes through to achieve better oral health.

Because I was so busy, I stopped seeing children, and I stopped doing endodontics. I wanted to focus on occlusion, bite problems, and adult restorative treatment. Further, I wanted patients to understand my practice was unique and different before we made changes regarding insurance benefits.

To make it obvious that we were serious about prevention, we implemented the Dental Fitness Program. This program engages patients in controlling bacteria and bleeding levels to prevent gum disease and decay. It objectively records past disease, current infection, and the risk for future disease in the same way a physician uses blood pressure and cholesterol screening to demonstrate risk for heart disease. It's experiential learning for patients and very different from a lecture on flossing. We maintain a historical record of their oral health to demonstrate if they are moving toward or away from their goals. Patients get a Dental Fitness report at every recare visit. It's comparable to a quarterly earnings report companies issue so investors know if the company is performing according to expectations.

During Mastery I had advanced consultation training. My immediate goal was to do more quadrant dentistry. But when I presented complete care more effectively, I encountered a new problem. Not only did patients say "yes" to treatment, but some wanted all their treatment done at once! I didn't know how to do that. So, I had to get more clinical training in occlusion and esthetics. I completed multi-year, advanced restorative programs at the Foundation for Advanced Continuing Education (FACE,) all the coursework at Orognathic Bioesthetics, Inc. (OBI,) and the UCLA and Pac-live esthetic continuums.

Looking back in hindsight I see that for the first twelve years of practice, I was in a high volume, high-stress, insurance-driven, disease care model. It was not designed to get people healthy. It was designed for a transaction--for repair dentistry to ensure profits for insurance company shareholders at the expense of patient health and at the expense of the dental team. It wasn't the model I chose. It was the model I allowed to happen to me. I believe it's the model that happens to many dentists UNLESS we take time to clarify what we really want, develop a strategy, and then take specific action to make it happen.

The five years after the Management Program were

transitional, building and refining the model and style of practice that I wanted, a low-stress, high-profit, professional model designed for patient health, and the long-term success of the dental team.

## The Twenty Golden Years

I like to call my last twenty years of practice the golden years. I worked nine to eleven days per month because I was able to triple my hourly production and increase profitability by 22% over the insurance-driven days. I took off ten to twelve weeks a year, six for vacation, and four to six weeks for continuing education. Overhead decreased to 50% and stayed that way.

We made patient health primary. We tracked periodontal health with the Dental Fitness Program, and we discovered that insurance benefits sometimes hindered their health. It was hard to believe. Patients were overly influenced by insurance benefits for treatment, rather than trying to control the causes of disease. It's like someone who is apathetic about a healthy diet and exercise because he/she has medical insurance that pays for blood pressure medicine or heart surgery. I wanted to help people make prudent long-term decisions and understand the importance of their lifestyle choices.

I'll never forget one patient interaction during a hygiene check. Bob was a middle-aged engineer. His home care was consistently poor, and we couldn't motivate him to clean his teeth.

His dental fitness scores made it obvious—it wasn't subjective or unclear. He needed treatment for new decay nearly every year. I remember asking him, "Bob, how come you aren't concerned about the heavy plaque buildup on your teeth? It causes decay in your mouth, and that's why you need fillings and crowns all the time."

He replied, "Why should I spend time brushing my teeth when I have dual insurance? I never have to pay out of pocket for treatment, and I can spend time on things that are more fun than brushing and flossing."

Other patients had the same faulty thinking—that affordable treatment was more important than controlling the causes of disease. But health is what really decreases the cost of treatment in the long term. Health-centered care recognizes the difference between optimal health and optimal repair. Optimal repair has to do with technical excellence. Optimal health has to do with prevention, behavior change, and helping people understand how they can help themselves. Dental insurance is a structure, a system, that reinforces quick fix repair or symptom relief. It diverts efforts from the more fundamental solution—controlling the causes of disease. In my hurry to treat disease (make money?) I had failed to allow time for education, motivation, behavior change, and lasting health to occur.

Now we handle dental benefits differently than most offices.

We accept all insurance and file claims for patients, but we assign the benefits directly to the patient. Patients pay us and then get reimbursed by their insurance company. As Dr. Schuster says, "You work for who signs your paycheck." If most of the checks coming into the office are signed by Aetna, Blue Cross, Delta, MetLife, etc. then the doctor has lost professional control and positioned him or herself as an employee of the insurance company.

It required careful planning to make the transition, and guidance from the Schuster Center during Mastery was very helpful. I got our staff closely involved in the process. Before the change, we worked to further improve the quality of care and service patients received in our office. We advised patients about the upcoming change for a year before implementation. We got feedback from patients' concerns and addressed them. We lost a few patients when we made the change. However, my staff and I felt it was in the best interest of our patients' health to handle benefits this way.

During the transition period, we established systems to monitor our progress. We tracked over-the-counter collections (monitored in the PMCR) equal to office overhead before the insurance change. Knowing the financial numbers of the practice gave me the confidence to make the change and know how to adjust to problems. Also, I had established a solvency account (a business savings account) that would cover my overhead for two years if needed. So, if we had problems, I knew I had time and resources to adjust and recover.

Thirty-six percent of office overhead is directly attributed to accepting the assignment of benefits. The fact that dental offices accept the assignment of benefits and have a full-time staff person filing and following up on claims means that the dental office is doing the work of the insurance company. Assigning benefits to patients is not a problem for those who make a commitment to their health and who desire preventive care. In the long run, preventive care and complete treatment are more comfortable and less expensive than ongoing treatment and repair.

Over time, the number of office staff decreased from eleven to four, and I didn't have to fire anyone. My team has been incredible! There's just no other way to say it. We facilitate some beautiful, healthy smiles for our patients, get paid well, and have fun doing it. Who expects people to laugh and joke when they come to the dentist? I would not have accomplished my vision without the immense support and talents of my team.

Lizette is the administrative coordinator. She has been with the practice for over thirty years. She calls herself the Cruise Director, and she excels at helping patients feel comfortable and loved. Joan is a full-time hygienist, and she's been with the practice for over twenty-five years. She is the ambassador of health. Once Joan cares for a patient, they won't see a different hygienist. Carol is my dental assistant. She's the short timer because she's only been with the practice for fifteen years. She has superb technical skills and loves direct patient care. Patients say, "Dr. Leary, you can take a break now, I'm in good hands with Carol."

The power of long-term, engaged team members is often undervalued by dentists. When I speak to dentists I like to ask, "What is the most powerful growth engine in your practice?" Many say technology, because their staff is undertrained, or their office has high turnover. My experience is that people are the most powerful engine of growth. But it takes time to develop them.

Our hygienist sees six to eight patients per day. I see one to seven. I used to see fourteen to sixteen patients a day. One patient a day for me happens several times when a patient chooses full mouth rejuvenation. It means I'm with the patient from 8 am to 1 or 2 pm. Then I go out for lunch and relax. I return after lunch and check hygiene patients while I work at my desk. Those days are what I dreamed of in dental school. I feel like I'm an artist making a difference, not a stressed-out mechanic patching teeth.

Our gross income and net profit increased, despite seeing fewer patients. Business books informed me that a third to half of the general population is willing to pay a premium fee for premium service and premium quality. I chose to focus on serving this segment of the population because most of them have a strong commitment to their health. They appreciate health-centered care and a strong doctor-patient relationship. They are more loyal to our office than they are to an insurance company.

When I decided upon this direction, less than four percent of dentists had positioned their practice to serve this population. For me, it was a good business decision then. It's still a good business decision now. It allowed me to practice the kind of dentistry I enjoy with people who appreciate my efforts. No matter where you live, there are always people looking for high-quality, excellent service, and a trusting relationship. I know colleagues across the country who have established this type of practice. I was willing to sacrifice some income for a better quality of life in the practice, but it worked out to be financially rewarding as well.

During the golden years, I had more fun, more profitability, and I did better dentistry. Further, patients benefited from better oral health and more complete treatment. I have three objectives for patients. I learned them from Dr. Schuster.

1. A masterplan of preventive and corrective treatment.
2. Accepting responsibility for health, and commitment to

controlling the causes of disease—harmful bacteria and harmful occlusal forces.

3. The opportunity to choose long-term solutions, not just patchwork repair.

My practice settled into a 60/40 split so that 40% of patients chose complete dentistry in a stable jaw position (centric relation verified with splint therapy,) and 60% opt for restoring their teeth with their habitual bite. Of course, not everyone chooses optimal restorative treatment, and that's fine with me. But everyone gets the opportunity to choose and to understand the long-term consequences, benefits, and limitations of their choice.

All new patients are referred by specialists or other patients. We average four to six new patients a month. Treatment acceptance for comprehensive dentistry is high so I can't accept more new patients than that or I get booked too far in advance and it conflicts with planning for vacations or continuing education.

In conclusion, the problem was NOT me, the staff, or the patients. It was the environment I allowed, and the way we were working! We were working hard to be efficient, but getting too busy, more stressed, and giving patients patchwork, repair dentistry. Now we focus on working smart, being effective, doing the right things for the right reasons, and helping patients achieve long-term oral health. People who want to spend their time, money, and energy away from the dental office appreciate what we can do for them. They finally get beyond bondage to repair dentistry.

After completing the Mastery program at the Schuster Center, I continued as a mentor and helped teach Case Presentation/The New Patient Experience with Dr. Schuster. I realized I enjoy teaching and I have a unique message to share with dentists and staff regarding the nature of health care and what it means to be a professional. Many dentists have advanced clinical training, but underdeveloped leadership and consultation skills. It leads to professional frustration when they don't get the expected return on the time and money invested in their training.

Typically, I teach three courses. The first is about how to free your practice and patients from disease and patchwork dentistry. It deals with how to transition a high-stress, insurance-driven practice toward a more professional, health-centered, patient-centered model of care. The second course is on occlusion, structure, and systems for complete care, and oral rejuvenation. The third is a health-centered hygiene course for the whole dental team. It focused on educating, coaching, and motivating patients for healthy habits and controlling the causes of disease.

There is a quote from Bill Gates who says, "People

overestimate what they can do in two years and underestimate what they can do in ten years." My story shows you can get started in the wrong model for 10-15 years, but it's possible to make significant changes so that you can still have twenty golden years in the second half of your dental career.

Here's the letter I wrote to Dr. Schuster a few years after completing the Management and Mastery Programs.

*Dear Mike,*

*I wanted to update you on many recent improvements in my practice and personal life. As you know, I had become stressed and frustrated by following the advice of various practice management "experts."*

*Wonderful things began happening as I started to implement the model of care taught at the Schuster Center for Professional Development. The problem was not me, my staff, or our patients—it was the way we had been working! We were working too hard to be efficient, getting busier and more stressed! Now we work at being effective and doing the right things for the right reasons. Some of the results are:*

- *Lowered practice overhead from 60% to 52%.*

- *Last year collections increased 6%, but **net profit increased 22%!***

- ***I now take off 12 weeks a year,** up from 3-4 weeks in previous years.*

- *$200,000 in solvency reserves, regular funding of pension for myself and staff at the maximum amount, profit sharing for staff, and no practice debt.*

- ***Healthier patients**—we can measure this now and do so regularly!*

- *Increased case acceptance--more full mouth and quadrant dentistry. I have had the time, attitude, and resources to take advanced technical training.*

- *Hourly production increased from $250/hour to $600/hour.*

- ***100% freedom from insurance—no Delta and no accepting assignment of benefits!***

- *Over-the-counter collections are 85%. Only 60 statements/month from 450/month in previous years.*

- ***More fun** and less stress and busyness! I see one patient at a time, instead of jumping between two treatment rooms and two hygienists.*

- *Improved staff morale and commitment—regular staff meetings and budgeted time and money for team learning at professional seminars out of the office.*

- *Some of the intangible benefits are hard to measure, but even more powerful—i.e., improved leadership and communication skills, and closer relationships with family, staff, and patients.*
- *A tremendous patient-centered new patient exam and Review of Findings process.*
- *A team developed a Policies/Systems manual describing our philosophy of care, complete details of office procedures, and scripted responses for common patient concerns.*

*__In short, I work less, make more money, have more fun, and provide better dental care than ever before!__ I know my staff feels the same way. Please share these results with as many dentists as you can. I am a missionary for the Center for Professional Development, and I'm always available to talk with other doctors about the program. I'm confident any dentist would get results like mine with the study and implementation of the principles taught in the Level One Management program and/or the Mastery program.*

*Thanks for calling on me when I didn't even realize how much I could be helped.*

*Yours truly, Tim Leary*

Contact me at twlysh@gmail.com if you have any questions, or if you'd like more information about creating a fee-for-service, insurance-free practice. I have a large resource of handouts, forms, and systems so offices don't need to reinvent the wheel when transitioning away from insurance dependence.

*Dr. Leary graduated from Santa Clara University, and from the University of Pacific Dental School in San Francisco in the top 10% of his class. He completed a general practice residency at USAF Hospital, Davis-Monthan AFB, Arizona, and received training in specialty disciplines of dentistry, including intravenous conscious sedation. Dr. served four years in the USAF Dental Corps, and he developed a training program for dental assistants.*

*Dr. Leary was in private practice in Menlo Park from 1981 to 2021. He was active in the local component of the California Dental Association, serving as President of the Mid-Peninsula Dental Society, Co-president of the Mid-Peninsula Dental Health Foundation, and Chairman of the Peer Review Committee.*

*Dr. Leary lectures on comprehensive restorative dentistry, and health-centered dentistry. He has completed extensive post-graduate training in occlusion/bite disorders, TMJ disorders, anesthesia, and cosmetic/advanced restorative dentistry. He served as a Conscious Sedation Examiner for the California State Board of Dental Examiners.*

*Dr. Leary and staff completed the Management and Mastery*

389

*programs at the Schuster Center (SC) in Scottsdale, Arizona. He served as a Mentor at the SC for several years.*

*Dr. Leary completed training in advanced restorative dentistry at The Foundation for Advanced Continuing Education (FACE,) the PAC-Live Advanced Anterior Esthetics workshop and the four-year curriculum at the Institute of Bioesthetic Dentistry (OBI.)*

*Dr. Leary is married and the proud father of two sons. His hobbies include cycling, tennis, skiing, flyfishing, and reading. He served as President of the Rotary club of Menlo Park and Menlo Rotary Community Foundation, and he led Top Gear, a leadership retreat for outstanding high school students in San Mateo County.*

# Appendix 1
# Power Shift

## The Case for Reform in the Dental Office

Charles M. Sorenson, Ph.D., and Michael Schuster, B.S., D.D.S.

We believe most dental practices today need reform. The reform we call for is a redistribution and use of power. Power in a traditional practice is vested in the doctor, where the dentist diagnoses what is wrong, presents what is needed to correct it, and attempts to provide corrective measures. The goal is to fix what's broken and replace what's missing. The recipient of this service is passive, powerless, and viewed as a patient. The perception of control of power, or lack of it, has taken decades to establish and is deeply engrained in the minds of the doctor, other team-members, and people who avail themselves of the services in dentistry. In reality, everyone involved believes this is the way it is supposed to be. Likely they are all mistaken.

## Dentistry as a Behavioral Science

Dental care is a choice. The fact that dentistry is a discretionary choice, made by people availing themselves of the service, casts significant doubt on the traditional use of power in the dental office. Being discretionary defines dentistry as a behavior science rather than a craft or sub-set of the medical profession. Few dentists or team members, however, see themselves as professional helpers and feel ill-equipped to enable people to make decisions based on their values. Thus, patients, in the traditional dental office are often disenfranchised. Because of the structure of relationships that go on in the dentist's office, patients lose their freedom to choose.

## Power Game

Due to the mind-set of dentists, team members, and patients alike, the use of power has become an elaborate charade. The power game goes something like this.

Patients come to the dental office expecting to be diagnosed and told what they need to do. They are essentially *powerless* and whatever has happened to their teeth since they were last in the dental office is largely a matter of fate. They hope that they will be given a clean bill of health, but fear they may not, and that it will cost them dearly. They know deep down inside they really don't have to do anything but feel powerless to own this reality. They don't believe it is their place to tell the dentist what they want. Instead, they choose to become passive and let the doctor lead. In most instances, they are provided with no other option.

When the dentist accepts the invitation *to seize control and power over the patient,* the patient, over time, *recaptures his power, usually by dragging his feet.* The patient drags his feet by saying he will think about it. Doesn't have enough money. Doesn't have time, and often cancels appointments, or no-shows! Often just says NO! Often the patient may ask how much it will cost only to say that's more than he can afford. Another form of foot-dragging is silence.

*The patient drags his feet in order to regain his sense of power.* This power structure (game) is played repeatedly each day in most dental offices. All parties dislike playing the game but believe it is their destiny, as they know no other game. Many dentists, I've discovered, don't even know they are playing this dysfunctional game. *(The majority don't 'see' the underlying structures that determine their behavior!)* Dentists, team members, and patients seem to accept the charade as a necessary part of the human condition.

Then, in the mid-70s, the power game (structure) began to change. Insurance companies entered the game previously played by two participants, and the game became a game of three. The patient, the dentist, the insurance company. Previously, the patient gave away his power to the dentist, now both the dentist and patient have relinquished their power to choose to the insurance company.

The disenfranchised patient, already feeling powerless, relinquishes his power to the insurance company to choose for him. *"I'll only do what the insurance company will pay for,"* is the cry of the patient further resisting, dragging his feet, in an attempt to regain power given up to the dentist, but now relinquishing to the insurance corporation. It's a LOSE-LOSE-WIN situation, with only the insurance corporations winning.

## The Human Condition

*We are all similar. Not the same, but similar!*

Each of us wants to believe we are without sufficient power in order to justify our behavior. We either believe we never had power, or we once had it, but was taken away from us by someone more powerful. The doctor and team members believe they are powerless to enable patients to clarify their values, determine what they really want, and act on these values. Thus, the dentist and team members resort to **'telling and selling'**. The patient believes he is powerless to choose on his own behalf, especially in the presence of a powerful dentist. Thus, he defers to the doctor, or insurance company to choose for him. This perception of powerlessness is fantasy, of course, but is learned as a way of dealing with feelings of inadequacy.

We employ special measures in order to re-gain a sense of power. This is called our style of relating. We all have a pattern of behavior that is determined by an underlying structure that was formed early in life by our parents, educators, and society.

*The dentist and his team-members seize power by telling patients what is wrong and what needs to be done to fix it.* Patients seek to give away their power to the doctor or the insurance company to become more powerful in the final analysis. Patients do this by deferring to the doctor's 'superior' knowledge and skill. The dentist's ego is only too willing to be seduced into presenting himself as the one who knows best. The pattern of the dysfunctional power game is now well-established. The rules of the game dictate that the patient gives away his power to the dentist, and the dentist takes it away by acting powerful. This may be called the 'setup' in the dysfunctional, passive-aggressive game patients play. First passive by accepting their loss of control, power, and freedom, and then active when they Drag their feet in various ways!

Patients believe they can regain the power they gave away, and more, when they **veto,** or **overrule, say NO** to what the powerful one tells them what to do.

This is classic passive-aggressive behavior. Patients 'lie in the woods' until a more powerful tries to exert control, and then, they trump his hand by saying NO! This seems to make them, in the final analysis, the more powerful one. The game has now grown to include: the dentist leads and the patient trumps and overrules, by Dragging his feet and saying no, by delaying, procrastinating, missing appointments, and not completing treatment. Often, by delaying or refusing to pay for services.

We like to blame someone we perceive as more powerful for taking our power that we originally sought to give him.

By blaming someone for taking the power we are seeking to give away seems to justify trumping his hand. We blame the more powerful one for victimizing us with his statements and telling us what we need to do. In dentistry, the patient blames the dentist for presenting an abundance of expensive treatment. This is seen by the patient as justification for dragging his feet in many ways. Blaming and dragging your feet is just another form of trumping someone's hand.

We like to blame someone for blaming us. The doctor feels upset and justified in blaming the patient for trumping his hand. He does so by defining the patient as having a low dental I.Q. The dentist begins to believe and says: "But you don't understand the patients in town. They are all too busy, or they don't have money to pay for dentistry." Now there is a stand- off. Each sees the other as an adversary. Both, of course, are mistaken. This charade is badly in need of reform.

*Reform must begin in the mind and heart of the dentist.*

## Reform

The truth is neither the dentist nor his patient is without power. Reform begins when the dentist chooses not to accept the patient's power which the patient is seeking to give him. This is the beginning of changing the rules of the power game. The dentist must **not** accept the gift of the patient's power but must choose instead to *leave the power within the patient's hands*. This, in effect, empowers the patient rather than seizing his power.

*The game begins in the beginning of forming a relationship.*

The dentist leaves the power in the patient's hands by actively listening to the patient's story. By actively listening for the patient's primary value. Values indicate what a patient wants. We believe there are four primary values expressed by patients in dentistry:

- **Esthetics**—they want their teeth, mouth, and face to look better, often more youthful.

- **Function**—they want their teeth and oral system to work better. People want to be able to eat and chew comfortably and efficiently.
- **Comfort**—they want to be free of pain, all pain.
- **Preserve health**—people really want no disease, but most don't know how to become healthy!

One or more of these primary values motivates each person to come to the dental office and seek help and guidance.

It is the responsibility of a professional helper to actively listen to each patient to determine which primary value/s motivates him. We believe that a dental practice must be a safe, transparent, accepting, learning environment. The dentist is educated first by the patient as to what the patient needs, wants, and how he wants to be cared for. The patient can then be educated in a safe, cooperative, learning environment relative to the causes of dental disease; the fact that dental disease can be controlled but not cured, and that dental disease, left on its own I progressive. The patient can be given the power to control her own disease and then allow the patient to choose the level of health (absence of signs and symptoms of disease) that she chooses for herself.

As the relationship progresses, the dentist and the patient discover together what a Healthy Oral System looks like *and* discover together the picture of their existing condition in reference to a picture of Health. (Contrast is the essence of structural tension) In this process, the game has changed from SHOW-TELL—SELL to a process of *joint discovery*, *joint diagnosis*, and *joint treatment planning*. The essence of this process is to help the patient discover and get what they really, really want. A partnership is formed. The patient learns to control and prevent disease and the dentist can protect, and rejuvenate the oral system to the level of health each person freely chooses.

Changing from telling to listening, from listening to co-discovery, from co-discovery to co-planning, is a process, not a formula. It is a process where the dentist becomes an advocate for, and then a partner with each patient, rather than an adversary.

In the process, both the patient and the dentist create a transformative relationship. Both are changed for the better. Both get to keep their power. This type of relationship, though rare in our current culture, offers us hope for a better future for all parties involved.

The type, quality, and depth of the relationships we create are the major determinants of our enjoyment, happiness, and success in life and practice. It is the single most important factor in your professional life and practice.

*The price of taking responsibility away from human beings!*

You can raise and care for your nearest and dearest. You can do your best to send them to the best schools, and best rehab programs, buy them the best condos, and never give up on helping them to have the best life possible.

But if you do so believing you can rescue them with your good ideas, your checkbook, or get them to live a healthy way of life, that mistake will make you both worse off than you already are.

# Appendix 2
# The 7 Driving Forces of your Practice

**1. Your Philosophy (Purpose)** – The deeply held beliefs and values that guide your life:

*Values > Purpose > Passion > Vision > Mission*

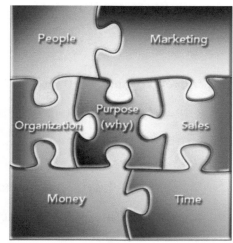

**The Seven Driving Forces**

**2. People** – You and the people you work with, your family, children, friends, etc. The knowledge, skills, attitudes, abilities, motivation, and desires of each person.

**3. Sales, Relationships, and Communication** – How you get along with people. How you relate to people and the kind of relationships you create with your patients and all others.

**4. Your Market** – The people whose values and goals are in alignment with yours. How you attract and engage patients and others to you.

**5. Organization** – How you structure your personal life and your practice life. How you deliver what you deliver in your practice.

**6. Time/Energy Management** – Time is life. How you manage your time determines what you do with your life.

**7. Money** – Money isn't everything, but your understanding of it and, ability to control and use it, can and will impact your life in many ways.

*"You need oxygen to live but oxygen is not the purpose of your life. You need money to live, but money can never be the purpose of your practice or life."*

Perhaps the most important thing I can say is this: These are the essential elements of a successful professional practice. Other types of businesses may have different elements and therefore different models.

Your practice is a system. Your life is a system. Each system is either alive, declining, growing, or dead. Each 'essential element' in your system is either enhancing the energy in the system or taking energy away from the system.

Dr. Mike Schuster

# Appendix 3
# Reading List

## Recommendations by Dr. Michael Schuster

<u>On Health</u>

*Become a health reader. The more you understand health, the longer you will live.*

**The Acid Alkaline Food Guide**, by Dr. Susan E. Brown

**The pH Balance Diet**, by Bharti Vyas and Suzanne Le Quesne

**Human Life Styling** by McCamy, M.D. *I gave this book to patients for 35 years!*

**The Pritikin Program**, by R. James Barnard, Ph.D. *I was on Pritikin Plan for 20 years!*

**Predictive Medicine**, by Emanuel Cheraskin & W.M. Ringsdorf

**Stress without Distress**, by Hans Selye, M.D. *Dr. Selye spoke to me in many ways.*

**Blue Zones**, by Dan Buettner

**The China Study**, by T. Colin Campbell, Ph.D. & Thomas M. Campbell, Ph.D.

**Whole**, by T. Colin Campbell, Ph.D. & Howard Jacobson, Ph.D.

**Forever Young**, by Mark Hyman, M.D

**Food, What the Heck Should I Eat**, by Mark Hyman, M.D.

**The Pegan Diet**, by Mark Hyman, M.D.

**Eat Fat, Get Thin**, by Mark Hyman, M.D.

**Confessions of a Skeptical Physician** by Tim McKnight, M.D. *Most ignore my recommendations for highly alkaline, oxygenated water.*

**The Blood Sugar Solution**, by Mark Hyman, M.D.

**Walking for Health**, by Mark Bricklin & Maggie Spilner

**The Heavy Hands Walking Book**, by Leonard Schwartz, M.D.

**The Wellness Revolution**, by Paul Zane Pilzer, 2nd Edition

**The Complete Guide to Fasting**, by Jason Fung, M.D.

**Dean Ornish's Program for Reversing Heart Disease**, by Dean Ornish, M.D.

**Stress, Diet & Your Heart**, by Dean Ornish, M.D.

**Beyond Illness**, by Larry Dossey, M.D.

**Recovering the Soul**, by Larry Dossey, M.D.

**Meaning and Medicine**, by Larry Dossey, M.D.

**The Enzyme Factor 2**, by Hiromi Shinya, M.D.

**The Dental Fitness Program**, by Michael Schuster, D.D.S.

On Creating a Life

**As a Man Thinketh**, by James Allen. *I read this book every morning for 5 years.*

**Motivation and Personality**, by Maslow. *This is the book that started my path of understanding of human behavior.*

**Release Your Brakes**, by James Neuman. *I wore out two sets of audiotapes listening to Neuman while driving to Iowa City from Dyersville for 3 years while teaching and in Perio. Graduate School.*

**Creating**, by Robert Fritz. *No question, Robert Fritz is one of the most brilliant people I've ever known.*

**The Path of Least Resistance**, by Robert Fritz

**The Leadership Bible**, by John Maxwell. *Without God on your side, what have you?*

**Toward a Psychology of Being**, by Maslow

**The Third Force**, by Frank Goble. *A layman's outline of Maslow's theory of human motivation.*

**The Road Less Traveled**, by M. Scott Peck, M.D.

**Further Alone the Road Less Traveled**, by M. Scott Peck, M.D.

**The Conative Connection**, by Kathy Kolbe

**Be All that You Are**, by James Fadiman, Ph.D. I s*pent time with Fadiman. I sent my children to his retreats.*

**Breaking the Rules**, by Kurt Wright. *A little-known but incredible thinker. Blessed to have spent time with him.*

**The Seven Habits of Highly Effective People**, by Stephen Covey. *Stephen Covey was a great thinker and doer. Privileged to call him a friend.*

**A Timeless Way of Building**, by Christopher Alexander. *An important book and a brilliant mind.*

## On Purpose

**The Power of Purpose**, by Richard Leider

**Passion and Purpose** by Marls & Merle Johnson

**The Truth About You**, by Marcus Buckingham. *Important to discover your Naturally Motivated Abilities. The sooner the better!*

**The Hero's Journey**, by Joseph Campbell. *The story of a Hero is everyone's story!*

**Answering Your Call**, by John P. Schuster

**The Purpose Driven Life**, by Rick Warren

**Preventive Dental Practice**, by Robert Barkley, D.D.S. *Most influential person in my professional life.*

**A Philosophy of the Practice of Dentistry**, by L.D. Pankey and Bill Davis. *I was fortunate to know LD Pankey personally and be mentored by him.*

## On Money

**The Richest Man in Babylon**, by George C. Clason. *This man's core beliefs transformed my relationship with money.*

**Think and Grow Rich**, by Napoleon Hill

**The Science of Creating Wealth**, by Michael Schuster, D.D.S. *A book I wrote in 2006 after 50 years of study, teaching, and application.*

**Money and the Meaning of Life**, by Jacob Needleman, Ph.D. *One of the most remarkable men I am privileged to have in my life.*

**The Millionaire Next Door**, by Thomas Stanley, Ph.D. & Sara Stanley, Ph.D.

**Money or Your Life**, by Vicki Robin.

**The Overspent American**, by Juliet B. Shor.

**The Energy of Money**, by Maria Nemeth, Ph.D.

**The Seven Stages of Money Maturity**, by George Kinder.

**Enough**, by John C. Bogle.

**Why Smart People do Stupid things with Money**, by Bert Whitehead, MBA, Ph.D.

On Time

**How to Get Control of Your Time and Your Life**, by Alan Lakein. *The contents of this book helped form my relationship with* *time. This enabled me to work 3 clinical days a week and have 2 careers at the same time.*

**The Management of Time**, by James T. McKay

**The 80/20 Principle**, by Richard Koch

**Time Shifting**, by Stephen Rechtschaffen, M.D.

**The Time Paradox**, by Philip Zimbardo and John Boyd.

**Gaining Control**, by Bennett.

On Creating a Business Model

**Organizational Development**, by W. Warner Burke.

**The Vital Corporation**, by Gary Jacobs. *Serves as a model for our students at the Schuster Center.*

**The Art of Leadership**, by Lin Bothwell.

**Corporate Tides**, by Robert Fritz.

**The Fifth Discipline**, by Peter Senge.

**Fifth Discipline Fieldbook**, by Peter Senge.

**Business Model Generation**, Co-created by 401 leading practitioners. *I was one of the 401 practitioners.*

**Systems Thinking and Learning**, by Stephen G. Haines.

**Developing and Managing a Dental Practice for Excellence**. *The 1<sup>st</sup> book I wrote. As timely today as it was in 1979!*

<u>On Relationships</u>

**Personal Power**, by Carl Rogers.

**A Way of Being**, by Carl Rogers.

**The Couples Journey**, by Susan Campbell.

**The Power Struggle**, by Susan Campbell.

**The Human Side of Enterprise**, by Douglas McGregor.

**The Professional Manager**, by Douglas McGregor.

**Bringing the Best out of People**, by Alan Loy McGinnis.

**Friendship**, by Alan Loy McGinnis.

**Reality Therapy**, by William Glasser.

**Choice Theory**, by William Glasser.

**The One-to-One Practice**, by Michael Schuster, D.D.S.

<u>On Sales</u>

**Process Consultation**, by Edgar H. Schein

**Why Am I Afraid to Tell You Who I Am**, by John Powell, S.J.

**To Sell is Human**, by Daniel H. Pink.

**Selling to the Old Brain**, by Patrick Renvoise & Christopher Martin.

**Spin Selling**, by Neil Rackham.

**Key Account Selling**, by Mack Hanan. *Brilliant simple strategy.*

**Changing for Good**, by James O. Prochaska & John Norcross.

**Instant Rapport**, by Michael Brooks.

**Truth Based Selling**, by Michael Schuster, D.D.S.

**5 Great Rules of Selling**, by Percy H. Whiting.

**Helping Your Patients say YES**, by Michael Schuster, D.D.S.

On Marketing

**Marketing to the Old Brain**, by Patrick Renoise & Christopher Morin.

**Successful Market Penetration**, by Mack Hanan. *Brilliant, simple strategy.*

**The Experience Economy**, by B. Joseph Pine II & James H. Gilmore.

**Made to Stick**, by Chip Heath and Dan Heath.

**The Private Care Practice**, by Michael Schuster, D.D.S.

ESSENTIAL READING

*Getting 'out of the box' of a traditional, mediocre life.*

**The Psychology of Man's Possible Evolution**, by P.D. Ouspensky. *Simple, profound explanation of why some succeed, and others fail.*

**Power versus Force**, by David Hawkins, M.D, Ph.D. *Life-changing theory. Be ready. Hold onto yourself!*

**The Map of Consciousness Explained**, by David Hawkins, M.D. Ph.D. *Written by his wife after his death. A far easier book to understand than Power versus Force. Hawkins was Wayne Dyer's mentor.*

**Wisdom of the Enneagram**, by Richard Risso and Russ Hudson. *The most important and useful book to read regarding the Enneagram.*

**One Simple Idea**, by Mitch Horowitz.

**The Miracle Club**, by Mitch Horowitz.

**Emotional Intelligence**, by Daniel Goleman.

**Spiritual Intelligence**, by Danah Zohar and Ian Marshall.

**The Theft of Spirit**, by Carl A. Hammerschlag, M.D.

**The Other 90%**, by Robert K. Cooper Ph.D.

**Grow or Die**, by George Land. *George and I used to have lunch together. His work on education and later, creating meaningful relationships is pioneering work.*

**What Matters Most**, by James Hollis, Ph.D.

**Finding Meaning in the Second Half of Life**, by James Hollis, Ph.D. *Hollis's work has provided a strong affirmation of the Schuster Center Model.*

**How to Want What You Have**, by Timothy Miller, Ph.D. *I've given away many copies of this book. Profound writing.*

**Psycho-Pictography**, by Vernon Leonard. *A new thought author with essential thoughts.*

**What's Your Point**, by Bob Boyland. *I've used Boyland's model to write books, lectures, and webinars, and incorporated his theory into my sales process.*

**HOW**, by Dov Seidman. *A pioneering book. Backs up our theory of human motivation and behavior.*

**Start with Why**, by Simon Sinek.

**Outliers**, by Malcolm Gladwell.

**Essentialism**, by Greg McKeown.

**The Power of Focus**, by Jack Canfield.

**Simplicity**, by Bill Jensen.

**The One Thing**, by Gary Keller.

**The One-to-One Practice**, by Michael Schuster, D.D.S.

# Curriculum Vitae Dr. Michael Schuster

- Loras College, BS

- Marquette, DDS

- US Navy-two years

- Taught Temple Dental School Part-Time 2 years

- Iowa Dental School—3-year Part-Time residency in Periodontics

- 2 Year Gnathology with Dr. Nile Guichet

- Completed Pankey Continuum

- Appointed Cadre at Pankey Institute

- Taught more than 100 weeks at Pankey Institute

- Completed Dawson Continuum

- Studied with Pete Dawson and Pankey Cadre

- Taught at LSU Cosmetic Continuum—7 years part-time

- Adjunct Faculty at Dawson Academy

- Founded Schuster Center in 1978

- CEO of Schuster Center for 40 years

- Completed Bio-Esthetic Continuum

- On Faculty and Board of Bio-Esthetics

- Practiced Dentistry for 52 years

- Developer of the Dental Fitness Program

- Developer of the Profit-Ability Management Method
- Author of:
    - Developing a Dental Practice for Excellence
    - Getting Your Patients to say Yes
    - Truth Based Selling
    - The One-to-One Practice
    - The Science of Creating Wealth
    - A Better Way to Practice Dentistry with Dr. Tim Leary
    - Lectured more than 1,000 days in the US, Canada, Puerto Rico, and Europe
    - Profit-Ability Management
    - Helping Patients Say Yes
    - The Creative Process

Received Pankey Hero Award

Dawson Academy Life-Time Achievement Award

Bio-Esthetics Life-Time Achievement Award

# Curriculum Vitae, Dr. Tim Leary

<u>Presentations and Course Offerings</u>

- Complete Dentistry Meets Occlusion.
- Remarkable Case Acceptance with Photos and a Compelling Story.
- Leveraging the Specialist-General Practitioner Relationship to Improve the Health of Your Practice and the Health of Your Patients.
- Looking for Health in All the Right Places.
- A 3-Step Examination and Consultation Process for Acceptance of Complete Dentistry.
- Go Slow to Go Fast, New Patient Engagement.
- Desire, Direction, and Devotion: a 3-D Peak Experience in Dentistry.
- The Art of Consultation.
- Esthetic, Functional Oral Rejuvenation, and Optimal Restorative Dentistry.
- Health, Freedom, and the Pursuit of Professional Dignity.
- Why Some Smiles Last a Lifetime.
- Mastery.
- Lessons from Peer Review
- Developing a Private Care Practice.

<u>Complete Dentistry Study Club (inactive since 2020)</u>

A 6-day continuum over 6 months co-founded with Dr Brian Mills. Training includes lectures, over-the-shoulder demonstrations, and hands-on workshops. Curriculum focused on:

- Complete Dentistry systems, forms, and protocols to support occlusal treatment.
- How to explain occlusal disease, and how to discuss the limitations of dental insurance.
- Create more fun, more profit, and more meaningful work in your practice.
- Communication and presentation skills to help patients want the treatment they need.
- Clinical skills to confidently diagnose and treat occlusal problems with conservative, non-invasive techniques.

<u>Education and Professional Organizations</u>

- Santa Clara University, BS.
- Arthur Dugoni School of Dentistry, University of Pacific, DDS.
- General Practice Residency with Intravenous Conscious Sedation, USAF Dental Corps, Davis-Monthan AFB, AZ.

- USAF Dental Corps, RAF Bentwaters Dental Clinic, England. Beale AFB, CA.

- Private practice of general dentistry at 625 Menlo Ave, Menlo Park, CA.

- Mentor, 2-year Mastery Course, Mentor at Schuster Center for Professional Development.

- President Mid-Peninsula Dental Society of California Dental Association.

- Foundation for Advanced Continuing Education (FACE) Burlingame, Ca. Director Dr Tom Basta.

- Pac-Live, Functional Anterior Esthetics, and Advanced Functional Anterior Esthetics. Director Dr David Hornbrook.

- Orognathic Bioesthetic Institute (OBI), All curriculums including Level IV, comprehensive full mouth oral rejuvenation. Directors Dr. Charles Wold and Dr. James Benson.

- Chairman, Peer Review Committee, Mid-Peninsula Dental Society, CDA.

- Co-chairman, Mid-Peninsula Dental Health Foundation.

- California Dental Association, Conscious Sedation Examiner.

- Duarte Company. Mountain View, CA. Presentation and Visual Story Telling training.

- Storytelling Workshop, Stanford University Continuing Education.
- President, Rotary Club of Menlo Park and Rotary Club of Menlo Park Foundation

## Non-Dental Presentations

Climbing the Grand Teton

Climbing Mt Shasta

Tour de Mt Blanc trekking

Alaska Heli-skiing